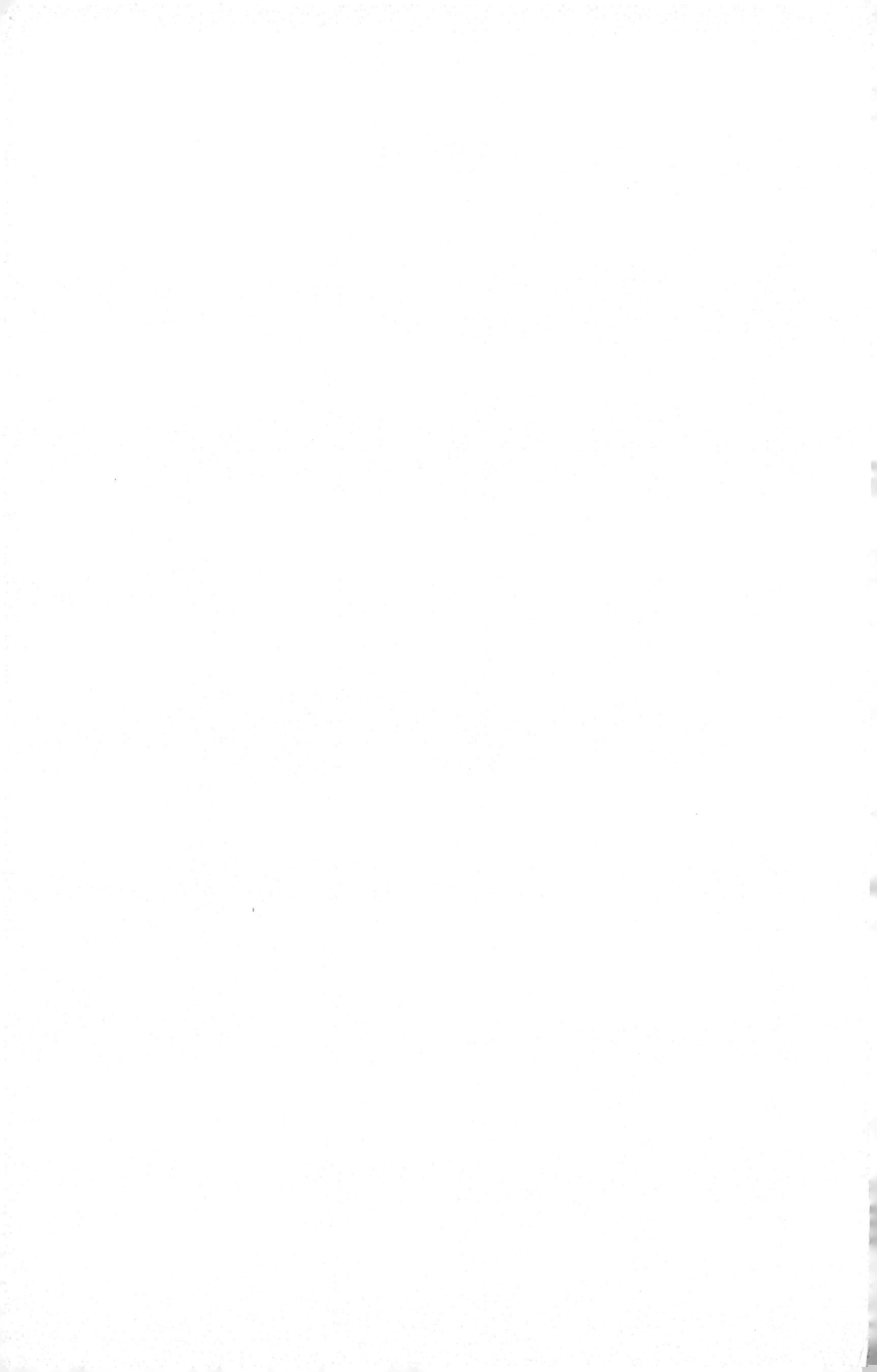

The Pain and Instability Solution

The Science Behind Chronic Pain Relief and Excellence in Mobility, Strength and Function

The Pain and Instability Solution

*The Science Behind Chronic Pain Relief
and Excellence in Mobility,
Strength and Function*

Dr. Michael Izquierdo

Copyright © 2020 by Michael Izquierdo DC, DACBN

All rights reserved. No part of this publication may be reproduced, distributed or transmitted in any form or by any means, including photocopying, recording, or other electronic or mechanical methods, without the prior written permission of the publisher.

ISBN: 9798554961380

Independently published by Dr. Michael Izquierdo

drmikeiz.com

Disclaimer: This book is for informational purposes only. It should not be used as a substitute for the specialized training and professional judgement of a health care professional. The author/publisher cannot be responsible for the use of information provided within this book by any licensed or unlicensed practitioner, trained in these techniques or otherwise. The reader should always consult a trained professional before making any decision regarding treatment of one's self or others.

Acknowledgements

When novel medical approaches are presented to the public, help is crucial to make unfamiliar concepts understandable and less technical. A number of people deserve well-earned thank you's for bringing this book into reality.

A heartfelt thank you goes to my editor Fran Kerg for helping me clarify, organize and elaborate the original thoughts and concepts behind this book. Fran, I couldn't have done this without you.

Thank you, Dr. Alan R. Bonebrake of Texas. After I spent years of diligently practicing, refining and discovering individualized idiosyncrasies within the specialty of Applied Kinesiology, our paths crossed and you helped me tie everything together. Your TTAPS course (ttapscenter.com/seminars), and invaluable mentorship allowed me to use all my prior learning and experience to see the body from an entirely different and expanded perspective. As you taught me, "Learn and put as much as you can in your head and sooner or later you will be amazed at what original healing ideas and concepts eventually come out."

In addition, I would like to thank my volunteers who graciously contributed their time and insights. These wonderful people are: Pat Lamb, Bobbi Smedley, Dr Lalei Guiterrez, Dr Phillip Belzunce, Leondria Johnston, Alice McGinty, Sam Lishchuk, Sherri Cronin, and John Myers, Esq.

Finally, thank you to my beautiful wife Melissa. You not only provided me with two wonderful boys, but your ongoing support allowed me the time and latitude I needed in practice to investigate, discover and fully understand the elusive defensive nature and tendencies of our nervous systems. Missy you are the wind beneath my wings.

Table of Contents

Forward 1
Introduction 3
Chapter 1: The True Cause of Pain... 6
   Pain and Pain Intervention... 6
   Getting to the Root of Pain 8
   The Activation/Relaxation Cycle: Balance is Key............................ 11
Body Connectivity 12
   Hip Stability and Viscoelasticity 14
   The Danger of Inadequate Pattern Resolution 18
   Steps to Fully Correcting Imbalance... 20
Chapter 2: FFF, Body Tightness and Injury.................................. 23
   What is FFF?... 23
   Deeper Into FFF 24
   How FFF Affects Structure and Causes Pain 26
   The Activation/Relaxation Cycle and Connective Tissue Breakdown ... 29
   Complete the Cycle, Relieve the Pain 32
   Anatomy and Injury 34
   "Freak Accidents": A Sign of Deeper Trouble? 39
Chapter 3: The Athlete and the Nervous System 40
   The Desire for Identity 40
   How and Why Training Evolved 41
   Body Specialization a Contributing Factor to Nervous System Issues .. 42
   Athletes and Injury.. 44
   Stretching Before Activity: Not Always the Answer 45
   Progressive Tightness Affects Athletic Performance 49
   "The Last Shot": The Importance of Flow...................................... 50
   Flow is a Habit 53
   Knowing the Limits.. 54
Chapter 4: Pain is a Memory 56
   The Optimal Nervous System 56
   Stuck in FFF 57
   Memory Pathways 58
   Cellular Memory... 59
   Neurological Memory 62
   Issues in the Tissues: The Second Messenger 64

Chapter 5: The Vicious Cycle of Pain 67
Scar Tissue and Microtears 67
Phases of Healing: How Microscopic Scar Tissue Develops 70
Small Muscle Atrophy 72
The Pain Cycle 73
Layered Compensations 74

Chapter 6: Reflexes Are More than a Tap on the Knee 78
Resetting the Nervous System 78
The Nervous System as a Computer 79
Reflexes and Sense Receptors 79
The Role of Nerve Cell Receptors 82
Ion Channels & The Sodium- Potassium Pump 83
The Nervous System and Reflexes 87
Understanding Reflex Reactions 89
The Positive Stretch Reflex 90
The Negative Stretch Reflex 92
Determining the Type of Response 93

Chapter 7: Structure and Pain: The Role of the Hips and the Kinematic Chain 95
Hip Instability and Body Pain 95
Deeper Into Anatomy and Pain 98
The Ongoing Pelvic Instability Problem 99
Muscles Protect the Tendons – An Unknown Truth 102
Getting to the Root of the Problem 103
Yes, Everything is Connected 104
Transformation for Strains, Sprains and Pains via Compression 105

Chapter 8: The Process for Practitioners 108
Focusing on the Practitioner 108
Assessment 110
Muscle Activation/Deactivation 111
Hip Stabilization 113
Balance: The Last Piece of the Puzzle 116
Pain During the Healing Process 121
Sports Rehabilitation and Chronic Pain Management 123

Conclusion 124

Patient Testimonials **126**
  Martin: Severe Back Pain After Playing Basketball 126
  From Sports Injury to Athletic and Personal Success 127
  Fayne: Great Results from Compression Belt 128
  Thirty Years of Pain GONE After One Visit! 128
  Alice Can Now Sleep Through the Night! 129
  Fifteen Years of Back Pain Eliminated for Fellow Chiropractor 130
  Fitness Buff Sees Marked Improvements 130
  "You Don't Have Back Problems" 131
  After Spinal Fracture, a Balanced and Healed Body 131
Glossary **132**
References **135**
Image Citations **137**

Forward

Michael Izquierdo, DC, DACBN has researched and is constantly developing means by which he can gain the desired neurological response to excite or depress muscular activity to improve function or decrease dysfunction in a clinical setting. This excitation or depression results in an immediate neurological response which can then be trained through movement and exercise to correct dysfunction and decrease pain and/or increase performance in a fraction of the time and with better results than traditional training and rehabilitation alone.

Mike's work with my patients, athletes and non-athletes alike, have allowed them to perform at higher levels without extensive adjustments to training methods or increased preparation time. Mike's system of specific neural manipulation and excitation, based on a patient's functional and clinical presentation, is changing the outcome expectations of his patients and fellow professionals. His results, in my eyes, show that the complex human body works in simple, expected patterns of movement and protection in reaction to injury, weakness, and pain. More importantly, he's shown me that the body can be corrected by returning proper muscular tone while retraining muscles that disallow normal function due to an autonomic nervous system that has assumed control as a means of protection.

I work with many professional football players, and my association with Mike resulted in increased response to rehabilitation and decreased time for pain reduction and return to almost immediate function. Mike's treatments have supported performance by minimizing compensation requirements of a healthy athlete's movement, because every athlete has some component of weakness and compensation which holds them back from peak performance.

-Jeffrey Lambert-Shemo, AT

Jeffrey is a Certified Athletic Trainer who has spent the majority of his professional career in professional sports and has had the opportunity to work with athletes of all ages. Jeffrey has trained and rehabilitated athletes participating in youth sports, high school sports, club sports, college athletics, professional soccer (NPSL, A-League, MLS) Professional Lacrosse (MLL), professional Hockey (CHL, AHL, NHL), Professional Football (AFL2, AFL), and also athletes competing at the Olympic Level in Track and Field. Jeffrey is also a Certified Personal Trainer, Certified POSE running coach, and a Level 1 Crossfit Coach. He is developing a track record of considerable success with older athletes, while continuing to treat and coach current professional athletes to enhance performance.

Introduction

In my holistic chiropractic practice, I've seen thousands of patients with chronic pain who have tried just about everything to gain relief. They have reported using massage, acupuncture, physical therapy, surgical intervention, and of course pharmaceutical drugs. Those close to me know that I have an insatiable thirst for knowledge and a deep desire to do the best for those who seek my help. Because of this, I have spent hundreds of hours extensively studying human body function, beyond what is taught in medical school, chiropractic college and most other post-graduation specialty courses. Fortune favored me by providing the opportunity to train under a number of innovative and brilliant physicians and teachers who helped me understand movement, neurology, anatomy and physiology at significantly deeper levels than most practicing chiropractors today.

This practical knowledge coupled with functional patient experience helped me devise a process to stimulate healing in the body that is efficient, rapid, and thorough by increasing nervous system functionality.

Once I began treating through this process, remarkable therapeutic outcomes surfaced. Equipped with a nervous system that was feeling safe, athletes suddenly became able to push past old boundaries and surpass previous achievements. Athletic bodies which had formerly shut down strategic muscles for self-protection became more coordinated and efficient, allowing them to push past their physical limits. Non-athletes who had compensated for pain by eliminating activities that brought them pleasure were able to resume those things that made life worthwhile *no matter how many decades they had been put on hold.*

You will notice that much of this book emphasizes the athlete and sports. The reason for this is because I love sports and deeply want to help athletes perform at their very best. I have a profound admiration for the amount of work they put into perfecting performance, and find it truly inspiring. I have worked with professional as well as student athletes, and understand how critical it is for them to get back into the game as quickly as possible, but with healing that is effective and complete. Rest assured that if you don't participate in a sport or treat athletes, you'll still learn priceless information about the human body by reading this book.

Please be clear that it is my firm belief that sports medicine doctors and athletic trainers are doing a fabulous job treating injuries and rehabbing players. In addition, I do not know where society would be without the advancements of modern medicine.

However, what my patients have taught me is that unless the nervous system is **acknowledged and satisfied, then** true and lasting healing will not be achieved. Because of this, the nervous system must gain its rightful position of prominence within sports medicine, athletic training, physical therapy, chiropractic, and every other body technique employed to take away pain or restore function. When the nervous system comes first, seemingly miraculous changes manifest quickly, not due to any Divine Intervention, but simply because the body regains core equilibrium and heals itself.

If you remember nothing else from this book, please remember this most important point: *The nervous system's primary focus is balance above all things. Balance signifies order, and order equates to survival.*

Whether you are a seasoned athlete or a chronic pain sufferer, know this about your body, *it was made to adapt.* If we could not adapt, we would not be here. Adaptation is how humanity evolved from lowly and vulnerable cavemen to the most dominant species on the earth.

Our human bodies are predisposed to accept most regenerative therapies the way a person dying of thirst embraces a cool drink. However, the nervous system will only accept change to the degree *it is not already preoccupied acting on previous survival instructions and mandates.* In other words, if already locked down in defense, the nervous system will fight change worse than a stubborn mule. You have to remember, whatever plagues you now, be it overly tight muscles, lack of agility and speed, stiffness or chronic pain, it didn't happen overnight. It has built up step by step over time through imbalance. Once the imbalance passes a certain setpoint established by your body, pain is triggered.

As you will learn, one thing people with physical limitations have in common is that they have lost the ability to maintain precise balance. Here I'm talking about a spectrum of limitations that ranges from an inability to move smoothly, all the way to debilitating chronic pain. In this book I will explain how restoring the nervous system to the highest state of balance possible eliminates pain, restores health, and yields amazing function and physical ability. As we continue to unlock the numerous secrets of the amazing human body, we will no doubt discover that all we need to do is to satisfy its need to feel safe and secure in order to trigger self-healing.

If you are a practitioner and employ the technique laid out at the end of the book, you will be amazed at the results, because the body will no longer fight you. By stabilizing the body and nervous system you literally hit a neurological reset button. Once brought to a new balance point, the nervous system will naturally allow the body to be more open to whatever therapy you specialize in.

One important note you should be aware of. You will find a good bit of repetition in this book. Hopefully you will not find this too annoying. It's intentional. There are some key things that bear repeating because my hope is that through reinforcement of fundamental information, the reader will gain a better understanding of how the body truly heals itself.

I hope you enjoy this book, but even more than that, I hope this information triggers within you a new way of looking at your body.

For more information on this work and to see videos of actual sessions please see my website at **drmikeiz.com.**

Chapter 1: The True Cause of Pain

Pain and Pain Intervention

The US Centers for Disease Control (CDC) states that there are nearly fifty million chronic pain sufferers in the United States. (Dahlhamer J 2016)

This is a large segment of the population. For many years, owing to a combination of social, cultural and political factors, many forms of treatment have been suppressed in favor of drug and surgical interventions, which were deemed in the past to be more effective, practical, or "normal". After all, if your insurance company will cover it, it's got to be good, right? However, now many patients seek "holistic" remedies. This means that they are looking for medical solutions that address their issues beyond the precise area where the pain exists in the body. They are looking to find and correct the root cause of the issue, not merely mask the pain.

Some patients have found allopathic (Western) medicine lacking or in some way not the ideal solution to control their chronic pain. I'm not saying that surgery, for example, is ineffective, but it's no great secret that many people fear it. Some may have friends or relatives who did not fare well under the knife, making them leery of taking a chance on a similar outcome. Some may have been given low post-surgical odds of pain relief that made them unwilling to take a risk. Some patients hesitate due to safety issues, because they have discovered that despite western medicine's affinity for clinical trials, few have been conducted on surgical interventions. The nature of surgery itself poses a number of limitations on how clinical trials can be performed. (Demange MK 2011)

As you are probably aware, surgical intervention is typically not even considered for pain management until chemical interventions (medicines) are demonstrated inadequate to control a patient's pain. But we all know people who refuse to use pharmaceutical, or even over the counter medications due to a myriad of side effects. And unfortunately, pharmaceuticals bring with them the risk of addiction.

According to the US National Institute on Drug Abuse:

> In the late 1990s, pharmaceutical companies reassured the medical community that patients would not become addicted to prescription opioid pain relievers, and healthcare providers began to prescribe them at greater rates. This subsequently led to widespread diversion and misuse of these medications before it became clear that these medications could indeed be highly addictive. (National Institute on Drug Abuse 2020)

The inherent risk of opioid addiction causes many patients to think twice before choosing this as a solution. Owing to the abuse problems of the past, opioids and other strong pain relievers are highly regulated and sparely distributed. Yet, every day medical doctors are confronted with patients looking for any solution to ease their suffering.

Patients desperate for relief often turn to over the counter (OTC) pain relievers, most typically those known as NSAIDS or non-steroidal anti-inflammatory drugs. These include aspirin, ibuprofen and naproxen. Common side effects of these drugs include nausea, stomach pain or heartburn and diarrhea. Less common, but potentially serious effects can include ulcers and bleeding of the stomach, increase blood pressure and typical allergic reactions. I am often shocked when new patients tell me how many pills they take daily, just to make it through the day, sometimes for months or even years. Many fully understand that taking large doses of pain meds, even OTC ones, have consequences. These unfortunate individuals are willing to take that risk, as they ask me all the time, "What other options do I have?"

Despite what's available in this modern world, it seems to me that there are an awful lot of people in this country living with pain who have been let down by all forms of medicine. Sure, these patients have options, all at varying degrees of effectiveness and most with some sort of risk. The NIH lists dozens of methods and treatment modalities for chronic pain patients to choose from, mainly chemical interventions. But you have to wonder, if any- or if even one of these- worked really well, wouldn't there be less than 50 million chronic pain patients in the US today? (National Institutes of Health 2014)

I admit that chronic pain relief can be elusive in my chosen profession, chiropractic. When I first became a doctor, my colleagues and I would see that some patients would feel great for a while after a visit, but then they kept coming back over and over again with the same complaint. Their adjustments would only hold for so long. This could go on for multiple years or decades. I was so determined to find the true source of pain that I spent many years after graduating chiropractic college searching for it. Hundreds of hours of training with some of the most brilliant minds in the country, thousands of hours of studying established anatomical and neurological principles, and feedback from thousands of patients have all brought me to one conclusion.

I now believe that the vast majority of chronic pain issues, and even instability issues, can be alleviated by satisfying the nervous system. And this can be accomplished in fewer office visits than typically required for pain relief.

Chronic pain is recognized by the NIH (National Institutes of Health) as a NEUROLOGICAL disorder. By designating chronic pain in this manner, the logical conclusion is that the nervous system must be addressed in order to make a change.

> As the experience of chronic pain is associated with activity in multiple networks in the central nervous system (CNS), chronic pain is considered a CNS disorder. (Chang 2019)

Getting to the Root of Pain

Can there be one thing in the body, one single source common to ALL chronic pain issues?

I have always known I was supposed to help people, and I also always knew it would be through the use of my hands. At first, I felt this calling was to become a medical doctor specializing in surgery. However, once I was introduced to the healing methods of chiropractic, I never looked back. The practice of medicine is an extraordinary and comprehensive profession, and I do not know where we would be without it. For me though, the idea of healing with the use of my hands felt perfect. In a way, I fell in love with the idea that through the use of one's hands, a doctor could release the deep and innate self-healing power we all possess inside of us.

Through the miracle of life, DNA develops each one of us from one cell formed at conception to living breathing individuals comprised of billions of cells all working together under the direction of the brain and nervous system in less than one year. I like to remind patients that if they were once capable of such transformation, the same wonder and intelligence is still alive within them. This very power can once again be harnessed to now make huge healing changes within their bodies. That mind reframe gives them hope that they do not need to resign themselves to a life of pain. The power within the body called the nervous system which keeps the heart pumping and the lungs breathing is the same power that can heal.

I explain to patients that when the nervous system is stuck in survival mode, it will not lend its full attention to healing the body. The chiropractic and functional neurological methods I employ are intended to progressively strip away multiple layers of the self-defense measures the nervous system sets up, and to allow its natural power to retake full, better and optimal control of the body.

Once I fully understood what was truly happening to a body in chronic pain, I knew that, as a practicing chiropractor, I would be able to help people while accomplishing my true reason for living.

In reading this book you will learn what has led me to the conclusion that the nervous system needs to be addressed whenever there's pain. If you are a chronic pain sufferer you will understand what to look for in a practitioner. If you're a practitioner you'll learn what you can do in order to help your patients or clients regain a level of comfort they may have been missing for years or even decades. If you're a sports trainer or coach, the information in this book can make all the difference in the world to the health of your players or clients.

Speaking of sports, you'll notice there are a LOT of sports references in this book. I'm passionate about pain alleviation, but equally as passionate about sports medicine. When I see a player injured on the field, I can tell immediately where their nervous system lost precise control of the body. This understanding is based on years of clinical experience seeing how the nervous system controls individual muscles and muscle groups. Too many athletes are sustaining multiple injuries- not because they need more training- rather it's because their nervous systems are over-worked and stressed out. When a game time situation calls for them to open up and expand the body for a dramatic play, the overly-protective nervous system will instinctively pull the "emergency brake," and tighten up as a means of protection. Tragically, the reaction itself can cause a player to pull a hamstring, strain a knee, twist an ankle, or come up limping in multiple ways. This is the fundamental cause behind most sports injuries.

Deep neurological imbalances often emerge when a game is on the line and the combination of fatigue and stress causes players to drop the pass, miss the bucket or swing past the pitch. If this happens regularly in tight games, but not during practice, this is a sure sign that there's a neurological imbalance. The good news is that this can be fixed.

This book takes you beyond the pain itself and into its true cause. With compassion, I tell my patients that I understand they hurt, but the treatment will focus on restoring proper function, and not on pain. This is because when the nervous system runs the body precisely and efficiently, there simply is no pain. Pain only exists to the extent that the nervous system is forced to cut corners and keep some parts of the body tightly guarded and other parts of the body partially shut down.

For a moment, picture the body like a factory with the nervous system as the management that keeps everything working. When everything is going well, the factory is fully employed and running smoothly. It takes in high quality raw materials, makes exceptional products and efficiently disposes of wastes. But suppose that, due to mismanagement, the system begins to break down. The inadequate management team must drive the factory to survive by overworking and abusing strained employees. Survival is the main goal of the management team, no matter what the circumstances are.

The body works on the same principle. A deficient nervous system cannot control the body optimally. But the better the doctor can help restore function to the body, the better the nervous system can work, and the less pain there is.

I am not a pain doctor, but rather a doctor of function in motion. The body is dynamic. Simply put, it is made to move. When the body is not moving properly, it is not functioning properly, and the result is pain. Getting things to move and restoring the efficiency of your nervous system is the true key to pain free living and optimal health.

The Activation/Relaxation Cycle: Balance is Key

For most of us, the days when we felt pliable as rubber are gone, but we should use those memories as the optimal benchmark for comparing the difference between moving in a neurologically balanced body versus one that feels temporarily loosened through stretching techniques, warm baths or massage.

I have experienced firsthand the apprehension and anxiety that both players and trainers feel when the athlete takes the field after rehabbing a serious injury like a hamstring pull. Everyone hopes for the best, but in the back of most people's minds lies the thought that the muscle, under heavy action, may again pull. For too long certain established pregame relaxation techniques such as innovative stretching or deep tissue massage actually set players up for injury and failure.

As a form of defense, the nervous system overtightens muscles when it fears for the safety and survival of the body. When these overly defended muscles are incompletely released through these techniques, and the player takes the field soon afterwards, chances are higher that the play will injure or reinjure a compromised area. This book presents a more effective way to release defended muscles

Most pain patients see chiropractors for issues from upper to low back within a few inches either way of the spine. In common everyday practice, other areas of concern include pain in the shoulders, knees, ankles, elbows and wrists. These patients often tell me that stretching and massage are no longer helpful.

To me, it's logical why these interventions aren't helping the patient. There is a tragic lack of understanding about common injuries and their foundational causes. As you will see, chronic pain and injuries derive from incomplete activation/relaxation processes.

Let's take a very simple example of this process. When you walk, muscles on the front of the body *activate* to lift the legs, while muscles on the back of the body *relax*, accommodating the muscles in front to allow the leg to lift. Stepping down with the foot reverses the muscle firing pattern. Now the muscles on the back of the body are *activated* to stabilize the body, while the muscles on the front *relax* to accommodate the action of the muscles in the back of the body.

To complete the process the muscle must come into <u>neutral</u> to fully rest for a fraction of a second in preparation for the next firing event. This indicates to the nervous system that balance has been restored to the body.

Balance is the essential secret to all human health. Balance is more than being able to stand on one foot. Physically, yes, the better the skeleton is held together, the better the person can centralize their body and stand on one foot. However, this essential concept of balance often takes on profound significance once one understands deeper and universal implications of what happens when the nervous system loses its sense of balance and equilibrium. When a player sustains an injury, it is not the result of improper stretching, but rather the sign of a body with a nervous system that's so out of balance that it causes instability. When a patient feels pain and stiffness, it's also a balance issue.

For the nervous system, balance is everything. Balance equals survival capacity. The more balance the nervous system maintains, the calmer and more ordered the body remains.

That's it.

Once the nervous system loses its sense of balance, it is progressively forced to make little continual adjustments in order to always maintain the best balance possible.

Body Connectivity

Within the body, everything has a purpose, and everything effects everything else through the physical connective relationships present throughout the entire body.

When the nervous system is balanced and stress is low, there is a firm but healthy elastic load tension connecting the muscles and fascia to the pelvis. In a healthy pelvis, the ligaments will be very tight and strong, but at the same time elastic.

Imagine holding a heavy work boot upside down where the dense black sole is facing you. In your mind compare that boot's thickness and heaviness to the sole of those running shoes advertised for superior lightness. The advertising sales pitch for the running shoes proclaims that the runner should barely feel them on their feet. When someone attempts to bend and twist the hard rubber sole of the work boot, the first thing they would notice is how it barely bends then quickly recoils back into its original shape. Compared to the work boot, the running shoe is spongy and easily bendable. Here is the point, healthy ligaments stretch and bend like a heavy-duty work boot and quickly recoil back to their original shape. Unhealthy and overly stretched ligaments bend like the super light running shoes, but unlike the running shoe itself, they are unable to return to their original elastic natural state.

If a person's connective tissue had stretch potential similar to the flimsy running shoe the pelvis would be extremely unstable. The state of calm and order the nervous system is designed to work under *is directly related to pelvic stability*. The greater the pelvic instability, the more the brain perceives the entire body as unstable.

An unstable base created by weakened ligaments directly triggers a continuous emergency situation in the brain. The medical term for this all too common weakened state is *ligamental laxity*. From years of clinical experience successfully treating thousands of patients, I've come to realize that hip ligamental laxity is the principle reason behind most of today's athletic injuries, faulty plays, and much of the chronic pain suffered in society.

When the hip is unbalanced the body will lean one way or the other. The brain will activate muscles on the opposite side of the lean to balance out the body. Instability on the right side will activate muscles on the left side.

Once engaged to fire for the purpose of keeping balance, these muscles will lock in place and the nervous system will hold continual tension. This is the area where the pain will arise, although it is not the cause of the pain itself.

Picture a tree partially chopped down on the right side. If ropes are attached to the left side and firmly held, they can hold the tree upright. Even though the real issue and weakness stems from the large chopped out hole which will eventually bring the tree down, the tension is concentrated in the overly-tight ropes on the left.

As you will read in later chapters, true healing comes from a process where control is given back to the nervous system in steps. Every step of stability and re-integration moves the body closer and closer to the nervous system regaining maximal optimal control of the body. In this way the nervous system operates the body from a greater state of calm and ease versus a state of fight, flight or freeze which is the innate survival response. The greater control the nervous system regains, the better it self-regulates and adapts. The better it regulates, the better the capacity to heal itself.

Hip Stability and Viscoelasticity

A major contributor to most sports injuries and chronic pain, is a core hip imbalance, and this can be the case even when hip pain is not present. Hip imbalance occurs when ligaments which are supposed to secure the pelvis firmly together weaken to the point where a person loses central hip stability and elastic potential.

For most who have practiced sports medicine or have otherwise been engaged in sports or pain management for a long time, this concept about hip instability may seem difficult to believe. The mainstream belief is that a course of anti-inflammatory medications, injections before game time, active stretching or pelvic muscle rehabilitation exercises will eliminate pain for good.

Body Connectivity

However, once the painful area is treated and discomfort is relieved, resolution of the problem is not always complete. In time the same pain and physical restriction returns to that area or another pain or injury arises very close to it, bringing similar physical restriction. Unfortunately, when athletes fall into this cycle, they lose agility and become labeled "injury prone." Non-athlete patients will at this point typically receive a diagnosis of chronic pain, in the hip and/or low back, and are told it is due to old age.

The spine rests on the foundation of the hip. The hip is made of two side bones and the middle sacrum. Those two side bones are called ilia. All three bones are held in place by ligaments.

Remember: *"Ligaments hold bones together, muscles move bones."*

Ligaments Connect Bones to Bones

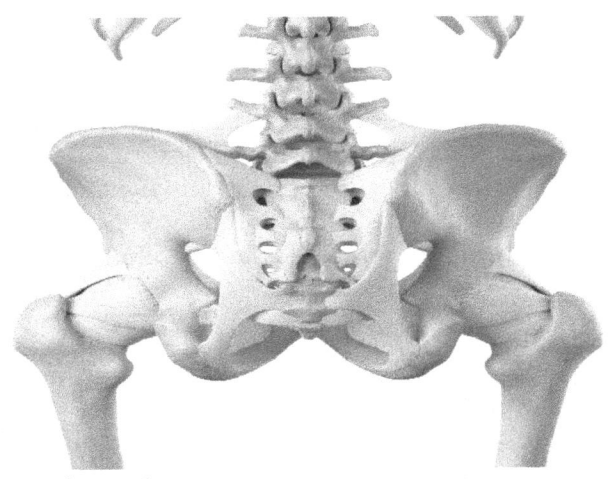

Image 1

The reason this point is important is because ligaments, tendons, and fascia are all connective tissues. Connective tissue is designed to do as its name says. That is to connect and essentially hold skeletal structure together. In connecting parts of the body, connective tissues have to maintain a continuous load or pressure placed against them at all times. These tissues have a property known as viscoelasticity.

Any substance which can spring back after temporary pressure, but permanently loses its shape if it's put under continual stress, possesses viscoelasticity. Viscoelasticity is often confusing with regards to the strength and elastic potential of the pelvic ligaments.

Let's get a better understanding of viscoelasticity's crucial property. Take any ordinary rubberized plastic trash bag you probably have right now lining your trashcan. As you pick it up notice the strength and sturdiness its walls possess. Now, observe what happens if you pull hard against a section of its wall. With strong pressure the plastic will stretch and deform.

You can stick your finger directly into the trash bag wall and push to the point where the finger deforms the plastic and your finger almost pops through. As you pull your finger back out, observe how the wall from that section of the bag is now dangling and unable to recoil back to its original shape.

Any viscoelastic structure once stretched past its limitations is unable to independently regain its original form.

The connective tissue that becomes your hip ligaments possess this viscoelastic property. When your hip ligaments get pulled past a certain point of recovery, their function of holding your base firmly as well as the ability to recoil from the shocks of walking and/or running is compromised.

If you suffer from pain, think about it this way. Your pelvic ligaments have turned into stretched out plastic trash bags. This means that under the constant strain of standing, walking or running, your brain will get the impression that the body is on board a ship during rough seas. The only choice the body is left with to keep the best balance possible against gravity is to tighten multiple large body muscles in a chronic state of overactivation to hold you upright. This continual over contraction brings with it the unfortunate side effect of inactivating smaller "finesse" stabilization muscles near the spine and joints of the body.

This is disheartening because these smaller muscles are the ones which initiate movement, coordinate balance, and allow the body to make very succinct and refined actions. These movements are traditionally characterized by words such as smoothness, expertise, dexterity, and natural artistry. These are the very terms coaches and reporters use when describing and highlighting the actions of star athletes, and this is no coincidence.

Remember, always, there are only two ways to hold the body together, ligaments and muscle. To the extent the ligaments cannot hold your body together, your muscles have to.

There are continuous muscle connections from the bottom part of the body all the way to the top. More importantly, various muscles attach and run through the centralized hip point from the top, bottom, both sides of the body, and even at diagonal angles through the hip.

Everything, in Some Way, Goes Through the Hips

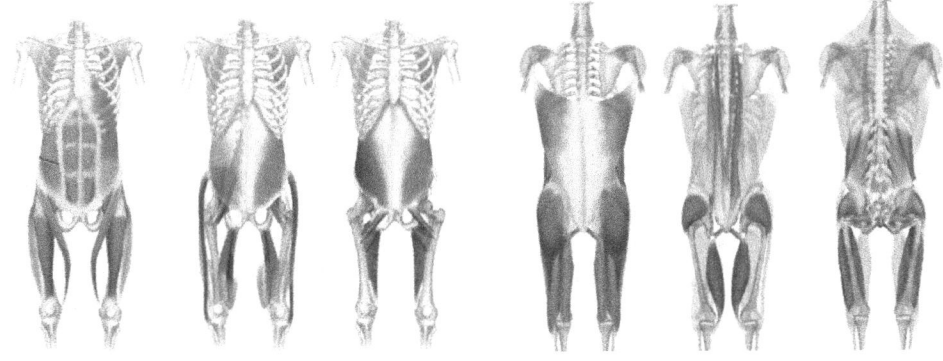

Image 2

Observe the picture above and note how many groups of muscles as well as fascia either connect directly to the hip or run through the hip. The chief aim of inserting this picture is to highlight the true interconnectedness of the body.

In your mind's eye, picture a spider's web. Now imagine which strand you can successfully pull on that will not in some way deform the web. It can't be done. The human body works in the same way. Everything is connected with everything else. The center of the human body web is the hip.

As long as the body is functioning well, and the connective tissue which makes up the ligaments and fascial muscle covering are healthy, the body can sustain incredible amounts of trauma and recover. The bounce back comes from the viscoelastic property of ligaments and fascia that are able to stretch and recoil *as long as they remain within their tight viscoelastic parameters*. The young enjoy broad viscoelastic parameters, which is the main reason why children, teens and young adults are so resilient. They literally bend without breaking.

The Danger of Inadequate Pattern Resolution

Psychologist Donald Olding Hebb pioneered the field of neuropsychology. His research allowed scientists to understand how neurons contribute to biological processes such as learning and the orderly neurological function of the body. Coined in his honor, Hebb's Rule of Facilitation states:

> *When an impulse has passed once through a certain set of neurons (known as the "facilitated section") to the exclusion of others, it will tend to take the same course on a future occasion. And, each time that impulse traverses this path, on all future occasions, the resistance will be less.*

This is typically summarized as "nerves that fire together, wire together."

This law is often overlooked when it comes to contact sports, but trainers and sports physiologists should take note that it is central to understanding the reason for so many of the sports injuries we see today.

Hebb's rule is not conjecture, it is a physiological and neurological fact. Every hit an athlete takes triggers an automatic muscle contraction by the nervous system as a means to protect the body. The more hits an athlete takes, or the more they exhaust the body past a certain point, the more the body triggers and reinforces pathways of survival.

Each defensive contraction produces *a memory of the environmental circumstances including the position the body was in at the time of impact*. Body position is an important aspect of the treatment and is essential in clearing the memory. This will be addressed in Chapter 8, which is directed towards practitioners.

As stated in the law, the more frequently a neurological pathway is stimulated, the less stimulation it takes for injured muscles to contract in the same way and with the same pain intensity as was felt during the original injury. Once injured, weakness makes the area prone to repeat challenges, causing layer upon layer of compensation.

Imagine a scratched vinyl record. The moment the audio needle hits that scratched groove, the tune skips and repeats over and over again. This illustrates the dark aspect of Hebb's rule which is the elephant in the room that no one in the sporting world wants to think about.

Outside of sports, most people rely on OTC and prescription strength pain relievers to control these chronic pain patterns. In most cases these issues are deeply buried memories of trauma the nervous system constantly tries to protect the body against. If these memories are released, chronic pain will disappear.

To appreciate the pain that contracted muscles cause, stick your leg out in front of you and tighten it as hard as you can. In about twenty seconds it will start to hurt and in about a minute that muscle will burn with pain. Constant and chronic muscular contractions are what causes stiffness and pain. After injury, multiple muscles can continually be contracted, at first of course this would be to a lesser degree than your personal experiment with your leg. This tightness, which is demanded under direction of the nervous system can lead to repeated injury and more serious pain.

When the body is injured, in time the area can appear completely healed. However, memory of the trauma will remain alive and well continually triggering and re-enforcing a defensive muscular contraction. According to Hebb's rule, this is why it doesn't matter whether an injury is current or not when it comes to pain. Pain buried as neurological memory can be activated and re-enforced by light trauma such as small bumps, pulls, pushes, or even repeating the same position the body was in when the injury happened.

Many athletes today are cleared by their doctors once injury appears healed, but they can still have unresolved defensive muscle memory patterns from trauma. As long as these memory pathways remain viable, athletes are vulnerable to injury. This is the reason why many athletes today are suddenly sidelined with injuries.

Steps to Fully Correcting Imbalance

Human nervous system reactions are instinctive and automatic, not intentional. Stress is nothing more than a force acting against the innate balancing mechanism of the nervous system.

There are three variations of stress: physical, mental/emotional and chemical.

- Physical stress results from an impact or fall. It causes the nervous system to tighten muscles to protect itself in response to the immediate trauma and it retains residual tightness to guard against further assaults.
- Mental/emotional stress causes body tightening in response, for example, to attempting to meet and comply with deadlines and expectations. Many people suffer neck and shoulder pain as a result of this type of stress.

- Chemical stress results from either exposure to toxic chemicals or the consumption of processed or overly seasoned foods. In this case the nervous system has to expend energy to offset any negative consequences created by the processing and digestion of these foods in the body.

Regardless of the origin, the outcome is the same. Muscle tightness, tissue breakdown, and the residual subconscious tissue memory of trauma are characteristics of all types of stress.

Maximal healing and restoration of optimal function takes time. In my practice with patients, correcting compromised areas includes bringing back the structural stability required by the nervous system to properly manage and move the body within gravity. Compensations are established in the body layer upon layer, over time, like the layers of an onion. In order to satisfy the release of these consecutive layers, they must be brought back into balance in the order in which they were integrated. Once this stability is reestablished, the muscle firing patterns must be recalibrated to allow the nervous system to regain exact muscle control over the body. Towards the end of this book, in the process chapter for practitioners, I'll lay out the steps on how this is done.

I want to make it clear that in no way am I advocating that any techniques currently used to override tight muscles are bad and should never be used. Not at all. Many of these techniques and muscle modalities are incredible, and should be used. However, the right technique should be used at the right time, and only under the correct circumstances.

Here the correct circumstances are present once the body is newly re-stabilized, and the nervous system firing patterns are progressively reset. Once this happens, the nervous system regains its ability to turn muscles on and off according to present outside challenges, be it during a game, or even in walking a straight line.

When the nervous system perceives the body as unsteady, muscle firing patterns function as virtual parking brakes, continually engaging to brace and hold the body back against danger. This is the reason for many multiple player injuries as well as uncharacteristic faulty play. Although the player's conscious mind may direct the body to extend and reach, their overprotective nervous system will either immediately tighten muscles in protest or keep their guarded muscles protectively constrained. Thus, muscles pull, tendons and ligaments pull or tear, and quickness as well as dexterity falters.

Once the body is properly restabilized and nervous system control is reset to a higher level of function then by all means use those wonderful and advanced stretching, massage and electrical modalities to override the muscle tension after practice and competition so that during periods of inactivity and sleep, the nervous system can safely re-calibrate to a new and higher level of function and control.

Exaggerated Defended Posture

Ask yourself this. How can any athlete perform at their best if deep inside the body their nervous system is continually tightening and bracing for an immediate attack? In everyday life, how can a person ever conceive of living pain-free if their nervous system is on guard and remains stuck in the belief that tragedy is right around the corner?

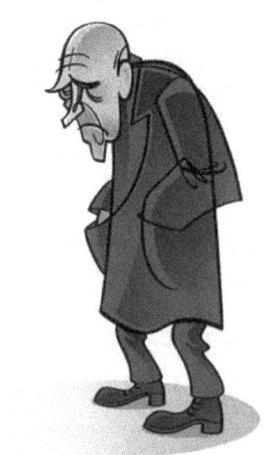

Image 3

As we get older, the generally accepted belief and expectation is that, with aging, comes overall body stiffness with an ever-increasing lack of mobility. That does not have to happen. When we regain body stability and reprogram the nervous system to correctly facilitate the activation/relaxation cycle, elasticity and freer range of motion are natural results.

Chapter 2: FFF, Body Tightness and Injury

What is FFF?

Imagine your cat Fluffy is peacefully lying in bed enjoying her fifth leisurely nap of the day. You arrive back home after walking Rex, your rather large Bullmastiff around the neighborhood. Rex can't wait to tell Fluffy about everything he saw on your walk and knows right where to find her. So he bounds, snorting his way into the bedroom with all the grace a chunky giant dog can muster.

Fluffy is not pleased with this rudeness, as she barely tolerates Rex to begin with. On instantly awakening, Fluffy is frozen in a state of suspended shock. One second before all this nonsense ensued, she was dreaming of stalking a slow fat mouse. Now suddenly here is this excited monster heading right for her. The instantaneous body-locking Fluffy experienced on first awakening demonstrates the *freeze* reaction of the commonly known neurological response of fight, flight, or freeze (FFF).

In seconds the initial shock wears off and as Fluffy regains her wits, she suddenly scoots off the bed and down the hallway headed for her special place on top of the dresser trying to find safety. This act of running away indicates that Fluffy is in another FFF response, known as the *flight* reaction.

As Rex continues the chase, Fluffy is hoping to make her escape into the next room in the hall. To her utter horror, as she nears the room's entrance, she discovers that the door allowing her to reach salvation is firmly closed. With amazing swiftness, Fluffy turns to face her tormentor with sharpened claws on full display. Within the blink of an eye, Fluffy hisses and leaps at Rex, slashing at his nose. This reaction is the *fight* response of FFF.

Here is the breakdown of what was just described. None of these reactions were reasoned or thought out. Perceiving an instantaneous threat, Fluffy's nervous system went on full alert. Her movements were totally instinctual. She simply followed an ingrained survival pattern established from the time she was a kitten play-fighting with her littermates.

The three FFF responses are all distinct and individualized states of being. Take particular note of how flawlessly smooth Fluffy's feline nervous system completely transitioned from one response to the next.

In the instinctual world of animals, once the threat is over, and the animal feels safe, the nervous system returns to a more quiet and docile state of being. With people however, many chronic pain patterns result when the human nervous system is unable to completely transition out of the freeze state into full activation of another FFF state. The freeze state is just that, a state where multiple muscles lock in place so that in the wild the animal has a better chance of surviving standing still and blending in with the environment. During flight and fight the entire body opens up to pure movement and action.

Remember, the FFF survival mechanism is designed to be an automatic system where the nervous system can successfully fully transition the body into whatever state is most appropriate for survival at that instant. Then when the threat is over, the body should be able to fully return back to a harmonious resting state. Although this is the design, the reality is often different, sometimes with negative results.

Deeper Into FFF

Faced with a dangerous situation, it's easy for most of us to go into freeze but not quite so easy to go into flight or fight, *especially if the nervous system is compromised.* The extent of each individual's adaptability determines the extent to which the nervous system can regain control and autonomy. However most adult nervous systems are stuck in freeze. Athletes make mistakes and get injured, and people are in chronic pain because an inner intelligence- like Fluffy's inner defense mechanism- keeps them stuck in chronically defended states.

Although athletes do not typically freeze like Fluffy did, an overprotected nervous system will continually tighten. But before I get into specific patterns the body takes when it tightens up, we have to go deeper into FFF. This mechanism explains the corner the nervous system paints us in when threatened.

In the wild, the best chance an animal has to survive is to not flee or fight, but to freeze right where they are in the hopes the predator will not find them. When an animal freezes in place, as long as they do not obviously stick out, chances are higher that they will blend into the surrounding environment, because movement draws attention. This is why a deer freezes in the middle of the road in the face of oncoming car lights.

Although the discussion of the FFF mechanism has up to this point focused mainly on animals, humans do the exact same thing. Think about the last time you were scared. Once your brain started to process where the source of possible danger came from, think about how long your breath had been held in, FROZEN. Police are well aware of the nervous system's propensity to freeze all body functions in the face of danger. Police and SWAT units crash in doors, scream, and use flash grenades to overwhelm suspects taking refuge in any type of structure. By the time most suspects come to their senses, officers can successfully pin them down and handcuff them.

It is critical to understand not only why the body responds the way it does to stress, but more importantly what occurs as a result of the nervous system's inability to reset itself once the stressful event passes. For animals, it is different. Picture a herd of zebras, happy as can be, eating grass in the African plains. In the distance a lioness stalks the herd. The zebras freeze in place and prick up their ears to sense where the threat is coming from the moment they hear anything out of place. The instant the lioness begins her attack, the entire herd disperses at full gallop. Inside their bodies the stress hormones adrenaline and cortisol are providing them with the power and energy to run for safety. The lioness will take down one zebra. The moment the remaining zebras have galloped a safe distance and realized there are no more lions, the stress hormones burn out of their system. They go right back to eating grass without a care in the world.

The human mind is so complex that worry about getting attacked, as well as concern for the consequences afterwards, sets up actual muscular reflexes within the body. For now, understand that severe mental anxiety before or after an attack immediately tightens the body and unfortunately keeps the body tight.

How FFF Affects Structure and Causes Pain

We all freeze, whether momentarily halted by fear, a quick attack, or even the joy of a pleasurable surprise. That instantaneous pause is the freeze reaction. When a person freezes, they naturally hold their breath in. Neurology calls this the abdominal compression reflex.

The nervous system's activation of the abdominal compression reflex serves two purposes. First, it sounds the danger alarm by freezing and tightening core abdominal muscles to protect vital organs. Second, once constricted, the blood that should ideally circulate to the brain and vital organs, can now be diverted to the limbs to run for safely or fight for survival.

One weakness all mammals share is that we have no natural hard protection for the vital organs in the midsection which is why the body shifts and compacts core muscles to guard them. This protective memory is embedded in the body tissues like information on a computer hard drive, and it only takes a tightening up of the body to replay this information. So, for example, when a boxer voluntarily activates the abdominal compression reflex to absorb a body blow, the reflex communicates a message through the entire body. That message is, "your life is in serious danger!"

When the nervous system is unburdened after recovering from a stress experience and the body regains its vitality, health and elasticity, ideally the body's natural recoil ability will immediately take over. As quickly as the core tightened, the abdominal muscle should smoothly decompress allowing the body to regain its calmer, and more natural and open body posture.

Without going too deeply into physics, Isaac Newton's Law of Conservation of Energy states that, "energy can neither be created nor destroyed; energy can only be transferred or changed from one form to another." I know that hardly anyone thinks of tight muscles like this, however the above point holds validity. The energy the nervous system invests to tighten the body up in its own defense is energy that is no longer available for long term survival.

Even though you may look and feel relatively the same from day to day and week to week, multiple moving parts within your body work tirelessly on a moment by moment basis in order for you to maintain the best balance possible. The nervous system coordinates that balance. Therefore, the nervous system will tighten and brace itself against anything it perceives as an immediate threat to life. The problem comes when this immediate safety mechanism goes on for too long because, when locked up, flow is restricted. Blood has to flow to keep the body alive, however, the full profusion of blood to all tissues decreases during FFF.

The biggest decrease in flow is actually energetic. When the brain signals any muscle to activate, an electric (energetic) current is sent to the actual muscle. When the body is stuck in FFF due to an incomplete, activation/relaxation cycle, electrical flow is constricted. An energetic impression of guarding is impressed upon the tissues, and this impression is held within the body.

It is this impression which leads to physical weakness.

Once you truly understand this concept, then you will share in my frustration at watching a sport and seeing players become needlessly injured. Many injuries can be avoided by correcting this hidden pattern caught up in the tissues.

To the extent that nervous systems regain their adaptive capacities, chronic pain typically associated with aging also becomes significantly reduced.

As it stands now in sports, trainers are dealing with pain and lack of motion resulting from the nervous system defensively locking up tissues. To relieve surface inflammation causing pain, or to stretch overly tight muscles only buys the athlete more time. When the nervous system is once again challenged on the field of play- be it through exertion or after a hard hit- the muscles will tighten harder and protective fascia over the muscle will constrict like a tight pair of jeans. Because many athletes are young and strong, this process goes through many cycles of tighten, release, tighten, release, tighten again- without causing the athlete any deep discomfort or concern. Once this pattern goes on long enough, multiple layers due to the FFF response become built up in the tissues until pain is felt.

One clue that an athlete, or anyone for that matter, should take note of is when they move from *liking* to stretch to *having* to stretch before movement. Another one is when massages move from a pleasurable activity to a required expense. The everyday stiffness athletes deal with and chronic pain patients perceive as a sign of getting old, is really a warning that your nervous system is stuck and is struggling to adapt. The more you are stuck, the tighter you get. The tighter you get the more pain you feel. The tighter you remain, the worse your body works.

Healthy and dynamic properties of the ligaments and all connective tissues allow the body to recoil back to a centralized and very balanced rest point. But continuous FFF incidents build up in tissues layer upon layer like an onion. Once connective tissues are unable to recoil the skeleton back to a precise centralized point, it is up to the muscles to do this.

Although by its nature muscle tissue is inherently elastic, when hip muscles are activated to perform balancing duties normally consigned to ligaments, they lock the body in place *because they are not ideally suited for this purpose.* The longer those muscles are forced to hold that position the tighter they become and the more they will enlist other muscles in this process.

Tight muscles, in time, will cramp. The fascia will activate and tighten around muscles to hold the best balance possible. For example, as fascia tightens, if certain locked down muscles are suddenly tasked with keeping the body leaning right to counter a left imbalance, over time the body will start to lean too far right. In response, the nervous system must activate a new set of muscles to counter this new unsteady right lean. And now a "snowball effect" begins. Layer by layer, the body gets stiffer and stiffer.

Unfortunately, most diagnoses and treatments focus either on relieving surface pain or helping to restore some degree of motion to an overly protected body. If treatment continually focuses on the first or second outer layers, then logic dictates that this is the real reason why many athletes, once injured, never fully come back to their full potential. Granted, many will get surgery, and do their rehab exercises religiously, but only a handful of athletes truly come back to their original brilliance. Although many may still be good enough to play, most coaches and fans' minds wonder how long this fix will last after bad injuries. For most it is just a matter of time until they get reinjured, or their skill level deteriorates to a point where they will be replaced.

The Activation/Relaxation Cycle and Connective Tissue Breakdown

We discussed the activation/relaxation cycle briefly in the last chapter, and we'll go into it a little more deeply here. Muscles fire to produce movement. But when a muscle fires, that is only half of an event. Like a shotgun, once it is discharged it will not fire again until the slide mechanism is pulled back to release the spent shell casing and the next shell is loaded.

When the nervous system is stuck in a state of FFF, certain sectors within chosen muscles will remain in a continual state of contraction. That contraction triggers local or generalized pain and causes the protective facial covering to tighten up like a virtual strait-jacket. This can strangle the muscles plus underlying tissue. In addition, blood supply and lymphatic flow may be compromised. I have had numerous cases with patients whose digestive conditions (including reflux, poor digestion, constipation and diarrhea) have cleared up just by resetting the muscular tone and firing capacity of the abdominal muscles.

Within these contracted muscles lie insidious memories of prior injuries, which continually trigger the nervous system to perpetuate the FFF state. Massage, electric stimulation, dry needling, rehab contractions and stretching are not effective with this all too common situation. The complete solution is not to rehab these muscles but to fully neurologically reset the entire affected muscle group using the body's own reflexes. This progressively takes pressure off the entire system.

Although a patient may pass the classic medical neurological needle EMG (electromyography) test measuring nerve to muscle signaling, deep parts of certain protective muscles can still be stuck in a chronic firing pattern. The needle EMG test runs electricity through needles placed along the length of a muscle in question. Any drop in electrical flow indicates a possible problem, but these tests measure major shutdowns *not minor imbalances*. These are subtleties within parts or sectors of the muscle. Remember, the nervous system's number one goal is survival above all else and it is always sacrificing itself to survive the present moment.

The key to resetting muscles and clearing traumatic memories lies in convincing the nervous system that there is no current injury to protect itself against. This is done by employing the body's own reflexes to signal compromised muscles to fully complete their contraction cycle and return to a more normal, calm and neutral resting state. To see demonstrations on how this is done see my website at drmikeiz.com.

To understand how muscles work together, picture a hand touching a flame. Of course, the hand immediately recoils. That basic recoil is accomplished through the instant activation of muscles in the front part of the arm. As muscles on the front activate, accommodating muscles in the back of the arm deactivate or relax allowing the immediate upward motion of the arm and hand away from the heat. Amazingly, the nervous system automatically coordinated and carried out this complicated action which seems very basic. However, if the muscles of the back of the arm did not relax and release, the biceps muscle on the front of the arm could not successfully move the arm and hand away from the flame.

The Hand Moves Away from the Flame

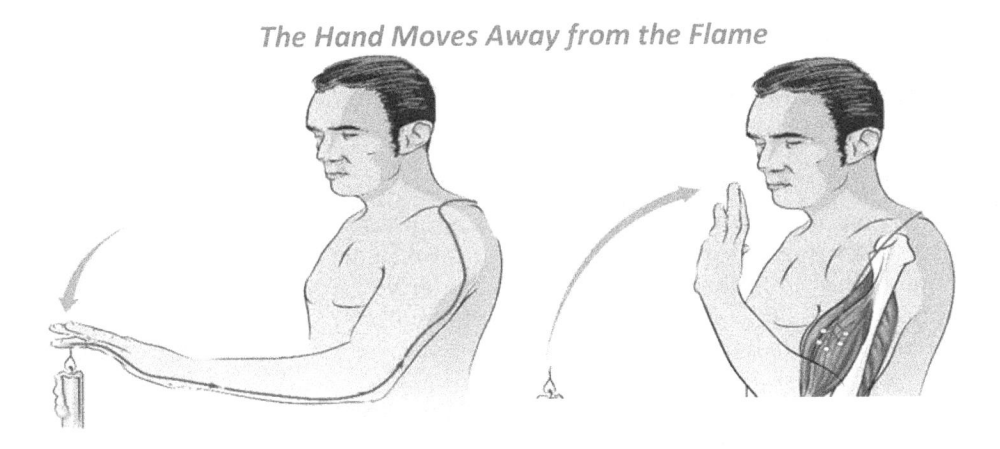

Image 4

Ideally, as long as the nervous system is functioning within a safe range, not overwhelmed or in FFF, then when the person lowers the arm both the activating biceps on the front of the arm as well as the accommodating triceps on the back of the arm will return to a neutral and calm setting.

The body is designed for movement. An incomplete activation/relaxation cycle on the activation side of the muscles is considered "trauma" by the body, and causes microscopic scar tissue from micro tears, sticking the muscle tissue together. On the side of relaxation there will be atrophy, because disused muscles shrivel to some degree.

And herein lies the problem. *Muscles in a state of chronic dysfunction can lead to pain and injury.* Pain results from inflammation. When muscles are constricted and tight, new false limitations are set up, and when stretched beyond these limitations they can tear.

The nervous system retains this information like a computer, so each layer holds a memory of the trauma that caused it to react. We will discuss layering, scar tissue and microtears more thoroughly in a later chapter.

Complete the Cycle, Relieve the Pain

Whether muscles are chronically contracted or chronically atrophied they have not fully completed their neurological cycle. Once I understood this, I began to view most common physical pain relief techniques and modalities from a different perspective.

Think about it, if lack of mobility or continual pain and stiffness is neurological in nature, how could massaging, fascial scraping, stretching, or strengthening a neurologically turned off muscle result in a long-term change? What long term benefit would be derived from using electricity to exhaust a muscle or even trigger point injections or dry needles which momentarily paralyze the muscle?

The fact that most chronic pain results from nervous system imbalances where the system has locked muscles in continual states of contraction was difficult for me to believe. But this is what thousands of sessions with patients have shown me.

Just as there are optimal parameters for heart rate and blood pressure, there is an optimal sympathetic muscle contraction tone of 0.5 to 2.0 Hz or cycles per second which is averaged out to 1 Hz. In many ways this pulsating tone is like a muscular heartbeat or a consistent pulse wave moving through the nervous system. Where the chief aim of the nervous system is to keep the best balance possible, the ideal balance set point is one where the skeletal structure is stable and muscular tone is optimally firm. This is the neutral stage which can also be called the sympathetic resting state. It's the ideal reset point where, once reached, muscles can successfully complete the contraction cycle. This state resets the muscle to a comfortable neutral. Recall the activation/relaxation cycle mentioned in the last chapter. Completing the contraction brings the muscle back into the neutral or relaxation state.

When it comes to physiology, Guyton's is the ultimate authority used by all medical schools and other professional learning institutions who train in healthcare careers. Guyton's will be liberally quoted throughout this book. Note what Guyton's states about the topic of ideal vascular muscular tone:

> A special difference between the autonomic nervous system and the skeletal nervous system is the low frequency of stimulation required for full activation of autonomic effectors. In general, only one impulse per second (1 Hz) or so suffices to maintain normal sympathetic or parasympathetic effect.
>
> The value of tone is that it allows a single nervous system to increase or decrease the activity of a stimulated organ. (p. 211) (Guyton, Textbook of Medical Physiology, Fifth Edition 1977)

What this means is that at 1 Hz the nervous system achieves dynamic balance. The sympathetic part of the nervous system is what stimulates the body to speed up mental and physical processes. The parasympathetic part acts like a break to slow the system down. At 1 Hz tone, the nervous system can easily speed up or slow down, tightening or releasing muscles as it sees fit, perfectly adapting to signals coming from the outside world. That same order is uniformly present within the entire nervous system.

Every part of the body is intimately connected. The order the nervous system commands is demonstrated in muscle tone. For an otherwise uncompromised body in a sympathetic resting state, an equal tone of 1Hz would prevail from the tiniest muscles of the arterial walls all the way up to the large muscles of the legs, arms, and chest.

Later in this book you will learn how muscles can be neurologically reset, thereby resolving incomplete contraction cycles which bring pain and constriction to the body. Each successive reset brings the body closer to the ideal resting rate of 1Hz. At this frequency, the body feels an increased sense of security because, released from an overly protected state, it can freely adapt to whatever the outside world demands. The closer the body moves towards the ideal, the easier it is for the nervous system to either speed up or slow down, and react appropriately to any condition.

From the perspective of the nervous system, any disharmony directly threatens survival. Ideal muscle tone cannot be maintained in an area where the nervous system is vigilantly guarding the tissues by locking down what it considers critical muscles.

In clinical practice, when a balance point is achieved, the result is obvious. Suddenly, previously tight muscles relax. As muscular tone becomes progressively restored, range of motion increases. Sometimes the change is dramatic, sometimes change happens in small increments, however improvement is always gained. As order is restored, stiffness and pain are reduced.

Athletic stiffness, which decreases range of motion, speed, and agility and increases injuries, is caused by layered tiers of activated muscles chronically stuck in contraction and/or inhibited muscles strategically shut down. These muscles are in varying states of functional atrophy- progressively made tighter by protective fascia "strait-jacketing" them. Inhibited muscles begin to take on the weak and shriveled appearance of an arm or leg muscle that just came out of a cast, but to a lesser extent. Later we'll go more deeply into how these layers are formed and why pain becomes progressively stronger over time.

Anatomy and Injury

Have you seen baseball players hit the ball, then round first base with a slight limp? Have you seen basketball players change body positions to run to the other side of the court and then suddenly start to hobble? Fans and coaches often are left wondering what could have happened. The next day, newspapers usually report these athletes have pulled a groin or strained an abdominal oblique muscle.

Growing up as a baseball fan, these freak injuries always puzzled me. Thinking it was "no big deal" when I observed this slight hobbling, I was confused at how something that seemed so minor was actually representational of damage that could sideline players for weeks or months at a time.

Let's take a quick anatomy time out. The end of every muscle converts into a tendon. Tendons act like hooks both anchoring and moving bones. When the body suffers direct trauma or you make a quick and unexpected movement with already tight muscles, those sharp and quick contractions put incredible direct tension on the tendons that are anchoring the muscles to the bone.

Here is a secret few know. *Muscles tighten in response to the amount of tension present at the tendon to bone attachment.* All muscles contract as a result of the nervous system activating them. As a general rule, if the brain is continually over-stimulated, the entire body tightens. However, if specific tendons come under intense strain, the brain will then tighten those specific muscles in order to disperse, pulling pressure away from the tendon attachment in an attempt to protect the tendon from ripping off the bone.

When a person's body tightens up from something like trauma or general overall stress, tight muscles place a lot of tension on muscle/tendon attachments. Muscles are designed to turn on, then turn off and then reset. However, in a nervous system that is maintaining a highly defensive posture, muscles are *already* tight and stressed and tendons are experiencing very high levels of continuous stress. As even more tension builds on those tendon attachments, the nervous system shifts priority by holding greater tension throughout the entire muscle in order to disperse the direct, dangerous and focalized tension on the tendon. I call this "weak link neurology" because big muscles will continually contract and constrict themselves in order to protect the tendon.

This state of heightened defense compromises the ability to bend without breaking. When continuous constriction is already present and a powerful significant jarring maneuver occurs, it can be adequate enough to pull tendon and muscle off the bone. This is the real reason baseball players, especially power hitters, pull and strain the tendon attachment of the oblique abdominal muscles partially away from the groin.

Whether the injury is listed as a groin pull or an abdominal oblique injury, it all comes from the same source and the same maneuvers. Until that area is adequately healed, every time a hitter swings a bat across their body, what they feel will vary from annoying pressure to severe pain. Worse yet, the nervous system will keep that area under constant defense, meaning muscle tension in that area will remain high. For baseball players this injury becomes doubly devastating, because not only are they dealing with lingering pain or pressure, the tension throws off their timing and disrupts their bat-to-ball contact precision.

Although the groin injury is especially prevalent in baseball, it is also seen in basketball, because these players are also rotating the torso. Whether they completely pull or just partially strain their abdominal oblique to groin connections, the resulting tightness and defensive restrictions this injury causes plays the same havoc on their bodies as they line up to make shots. Now that you are aware of this process, you can hopefully see how this affects athletes across the full spectrum of sports. This includes the golfer attempting to hit a power shot off the tee, the hockey player attempting to hit a slap shot, and a karate blackbelt torqueing their body to deliver a spinning roundhouse or back kick.

Abdominal Obliques Connecting to Ribs

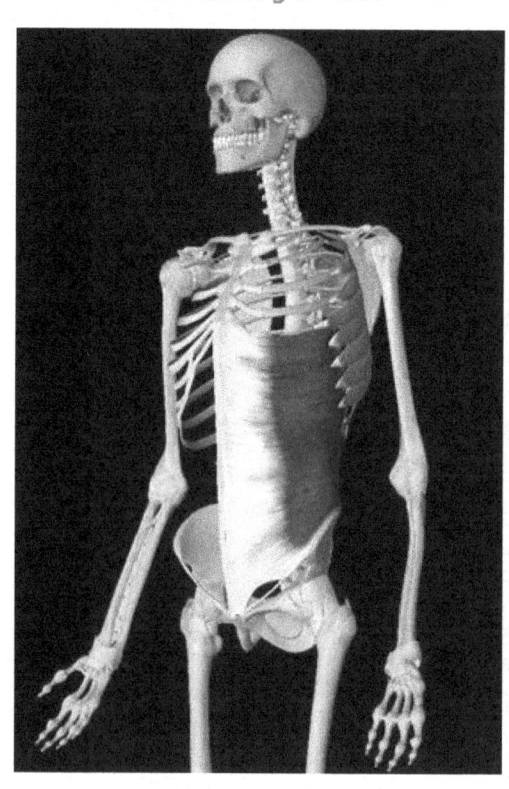

Image 5

Traditionally, oblique injuries are taken at face value by many trainers, doctors and therapists. This means that once diagnosed with a groin or abdominal muscle pull, conventional therapy dictates that the inflammation control and rehab should focus only on where it hurts, not on what I have found to be its true origin. Once firm contact of the tendon to the bone is reestablished, range of motion has improved and an acceptable degree of strength has returned, most athletes are medically cleared to resume their previous activity.

Before you fall into the above trap, take a good look at this picture. Consider how the nervous system activates long chains of muscles and fascia to stabilize the body while mandating coordinated movement. Note what the abdominal oblique muscles look like. Pay attention to the way its origin attaches at the front pelvic groin, and how it moves diagonally across that side of the torso ending at attachment sites along ribs 5 through 12. As a reference point, the 5th rib is located at the height of the nipple. Now examine the overlapping anterior serratus muscle hugging the ribs and landing at a junction point with the abdominal obliques on ribs 5 through 9. There's an overlap of the abdominal oblique and the serratus anterior muscle which looks like a staircase along the ribs ending underneath the arm.

The anterior serratus, besides helping to elevate the ribs when breathing, also lowers the arm from a raised position as well as brings the shoulder blade internally and forward. Imagine a baseball batter standing in the ready position about to swing at a pitch, the anterior serratus steadies the backside shoulder and bent raised arm.

The reason why groin pulls are so serious in sports involving significant torso rotation is because of their interlinking nature. The obliques attach from ribs 5 through 12, and the anterior serratus attaches from ribs 1 through 9. The overlap at ribs 5 to 9 creates what's called the kinematic chain. The kinematic chain acts as a rope of muscles connecting the body from armpit to groin as one muscular unit. We will discuss the kinematic chain again later in the book so you can gain a deeper understanding of its role in structure. The moment a batter attempts to hit a ball, their front foot steps forward. The kinematic chain is designed to work as one unit to transfer the power wave from the foot that steps forward to the shin (anterior tibialis) to the quads transitioning to the thigh muscles (adductors), and the groin. That frontward leg thrust triggers the huge abdominal oblique to rotate the torso to turn the body. Before the torso fully rotates, that momentum then activates the anterior serratus to start and continue the rotary motion by stabilizing the shoulder while driving it

Kinematic Muscle Chain

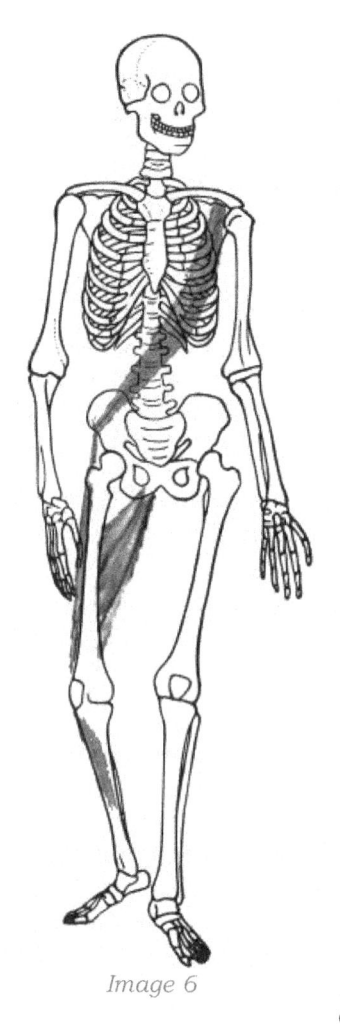

inwards and forward, as the bat traverses the full length of the body. At the groin the hips rotate, continuing a wave of motion through the shoulder, out the arms, and finally through the head of the bat.

With a significant injury, intense pain results with every swing. However, what if there is only minimal strain at the groin -- one where focused stretching and massage makes the area feel decent enough to play? Here, a groin injury is more than just a groin injury. Any imbalance at any place in the kinematic chain will throw off the precise timing of the swing or coordination. Players know when they feel "off", and coaches see it live or when they break down the swinging motion on film. The point is, this is not just a groin discomfort, it is the very essential essence of body balance and athletic mechanics.

Now take a close look at this picture and note the kinematic chain that goes from the groin to the armpit.

A strain in the shoulder stemming from trauma to the upper arm or shoulder area could be a hidden factor creating varying degrees of consistent muscle contractions from the anterior serratus, down the abdominal obliques and into the groin. Since we are dealing with a continuous kinematic muscular chain, this groin imbalance could also create tight and restricted shoulder mobility.

Image 6

Now you can understand how a shoulder or even a knee injury can occur after a player strained a groin or abdominal oblique muscle.

In a baseball player this condition would present with the athlete losing velocity or distance in their throwing ability because muscles at the armpit would remain continually tight. Oftentimes, this muscle attachment from the hip to the opposite shoulder is the true cause of freak shoulder injuries occurring after groin pulls.

"Freak Accidents": A Sign of Deeper Trouble?

In the case of a power hitter suddenly having to leave a game because of a sudden pull, their last fateful bat swing was probably just the tip of the iceberg. Lurking deep under the surface lay months, if not years of small defensive compensations that, like trickles of water collecting in a cup, finally overflowed. Most "random" sports accidents are not random at all, but rather a result of many layers which during one fateful "at bat" overwhelmed the nervous system's ability to maintain dynamic balance. At that moment the player's body is usually weighed down with a culmination of multiple levels of stress. This can be called "compensation layering".

Through functional neurological testing procedures, thousands of clinical patients have proven to me that this layering phenomena is the causative factor behind many of these supposed freak accidents as well as many cases of chronic pain and body tightness.

For those not convinced of the presence of layering, here's more information. A professional baseball player's body is conditioned through years of playing to rotate their torso powerfully while swinging a bat. According to "use it or lose it" training logic, during the season the player's body is supposedly in great shape and they have swung the bat enough times that an oblique abdominal pull should never happen. However, the unfortunate truth is that this type of twisting injury happens all the time, not only in baseball but in a diverse spectrum of sports. If it is not a layering effect coming to an uncontrollable head, then what could it be?

Chapter 3: The Athlete and the Nervous System

The Desire for Identity

In this chapter I want to cover a couple points of importance in regards to sports when considering the nervous system's effect on the athlete. Specifically, we will be looking at changes in player physicality, training, and flow.

Some critics have argued that sports programs are a waste of time and money, while others advocate that certain contact sports should be banned due to the increased rate of injuries now commonly observed in modern sports. Although every specific argument possesses some truth, the point is that sports epitomizes man's struggle to survive and thrive.

Although humanity must overcome the elements, predators and rival groups, deep within the heart of every person lies the yearning for a special identity- the desire for a meaningful life. People challenge themselves to grow strong or agile enough to overcome environmental challenges, like rock climbing or running long distances. In groups, people challenge each other to establish dominance and pecking order within the group.

Sports represent more than box scores and championships. This microcosm of life symbolizes the natural inclination we all carry within to challenge ourselves as well as push the boundary of perceived limits.

The calmer the nervous system remains, the greater the chance of success. It makes no difference if goals are in regards to personal achievement, or within the confines of teamwork. The nervous system, once properly harnessed, will allow athletes to enter and remain in the flow, paving the way for higher accomplishments.

How and Why Training Evolved

Athletes are in a new world today due to the intensity and the advancement of modern training methods. These training progressions push the body so hard that athletes walk a tightrope between overcoming adversity to gain strength, and locking the body into FFF by overwhelming the nervous system.

Why is all this intense training and action taking place? Because of the money involved. Professional athletes are an expensive commodity that require a lot of upkeep. But this wasn't always the case.

Bill Lubinger of the Cleveland Plain Dealer wrote an interesting article titled "Remember when … off-season was work time for the Cleveland Browns (and all pro athletes)?." (Lubinger 2019) In it he relates that during the early years of sports it was common for pro athletes to take jobs or run businesses on the side to supplement incomes from their professional careers. Back then, most players essentially earned a working man's salary. Star players like the legendary Cleveland Brown's fullback Jim Brown, during the 1960's was one of the highest paid players earning $85,000.00 per year. Compare that to the 2020 Super Bowl's Most Valuable Player, Patrick Mahomes' new contract extension. Playing quarterback for the Kansas City Chiefs, the organization sought to both reward him for his outstanding play as well as lock him into a long-term contract. According to Chiefswire.usatoday.com, Mahomes agreed to a ten-year extension that along with incentives is worth a total of $503 million dollars. Structured over ten years, his 2020 base salary is $825,000 plus he received a signing bonus of $4,521,508.00. Each year his base salary increases until by 2031 it maxes out at $38,000,000 per season. (Goldman 2020)

Lubinger's article relates how Steve Sabol of NFL Films remembers that when he interviewed star receiver Raymond Berry of the Baltimore Colts in the early 1960s, they talked about how the great Baltimore quarterback Johnny Unitas once laid linoleum on Berry's floor. During those early years of football, athletes would arrive at training camp to train and prepare their bodies for the rigors of the season. The off time between seasons allowed the body to heal and the nervous system to reset. According to new modern standards, however, that extended rest took away from continual training to keep the body perpetually strong and powerful.

Today, thanks to the astronomical rise in salaries, professional athletes are encouraged to train continuously through their off-seasons. On paper this strategy of continual training makes sense. However, this behavior brings with it a drawback. Refusing to allow the body to rest keeps neurological patterns and memories of trauma and FFF fresh within the nervous system pathways.

Body Specialization a Contributing Factor to Nervous System Issues

One important distinguishing factor that must be addressed is the dramatic difference between today's athletes versus those in the past. According to my colleague and head trainer for the Cleveland Gladiators of the Arena Football League, Jeff Lambert Shemo, one major reason for so many athletic injuries today versus yesteryear is because today's athletes are simply more powerful than in the past.

Shemo possesses over twenty years' experience working with professional athletes at all levels. According to Shemo, today's average player would be considered on par with yesteryear's standout players. Modern players are bigger, stronger and faster.

Collisions by contemporary athletes have literally surpassed the human body's capacity to properly absorb, adapt and fully recover. Today they have become so violent that this literally forced football to change. New rules govern how players tackle, with helmet to helmet collisions no longer permitted. Even with these new guidelines, competitive sports impacts are inevitable. All sports in some form or fashion traumatize the nervous system and force it to maintain varying scale of FFF, forcing the body to continually maintain a tight overall muscular tone. In this way the athlete is already braced for the next collision. The focus of this book in no way advocates less contact and greater passivity, which of course would never happen as it would make competition less exciting.

The key lies in successfully resetting the nervous system, paving the way for greater recovery, better play, and less injuries.

Note for yourself the differences. During the 1920's, most football players were roughly the same size. Although players got taller over years, it wasn't until the late 1970's that body specialization started to really take form due to football's rise in popularity and the dramatic escalations in player salaries.

By 2014, the era of specialization hit full force. Football had evolved into choosing certain body types, and training athletes to best serve their positions. For instance, cornerback defenders are characteristically short and light providing a lower center of gravity to run backwards defending their assigned receivers. By comparison, wide receivers are typically tall and lanky giving them the ability to out-jump the defender and snatch the ball at its highest point.

The most dramatic overall change took place in the 1980's with the rise of the jumbo lineman. During the 20's these players averaged 6 feet in height and weighed around 210 pounds. From 1970 to now the average offensive lineman grew in height from between 6'4" to 6'5" and weight from 270 to over 300 pounds.   (NFL Football Operations 2015)

Football lineman of today are no longer considered the slow "fat boys." They are now markedly muscle bound and considerably faster than linemen of the past. These athletes are highly trained, extremely conditioned and incredibly powerful. A good portion of their weight is made up of strong, dense muscle, which I learned firsthand when adjusting the Cleveland Gladiators. When these players get a head of steam and momentum behind them, whoever they hit definitely feels it. Unfortunately, there is only so much the body can take. Quarterbacks are in no way fragile. The general public can only imagine how much force a 300-pound defensive lineman generates when his entire body lands on a quarterback , who is focused on passing the ball downfield, and not on taking a hit. The body has its limitations, and ribs, collarbones and bendable joints are more vulnerable than assumed by many.

Today pro sports finds itself at a crossroads. Up until this point if an athlete wanted to improve, the solution was to work out harder. But now athletes have grown so immense and performance training has gotten so advanced, that according to some experienced athletic trainers, the body is fast reaching its limit in the ability to recover from punishment.

To say the solution is to avoid further and more severe injuries lies in more specialized or more intense strength training is ludicrous. How much further can trainers strengthen athlete's bodies against force impact injuries? There are definite limits to human physiology.

Let's face the reality of the situation that sports and the money behind it has created. Intense training will continue and even surpass the current pace it is in. Athletes will continue to grow stronger and more powerful. But the body can only handle so much punishment. From a neurological standpoint, as it stands, most of today's athletes are not able to fully recover and regain optimal dexterity. After each injury and rehab assignment, most players are just a little tighter than before. Although still able to play, too many high-level athletes are just not the same. The reason is not due to age, it's due to the buildup of progressive layers of compensation the nervous system had to take on, impact by impact in order to continually defend itself.

Athletes and Injury

In stadiums and arenas across the country, college and professional athletes are suffering needless injuries. When stars go down, sports analysts usually blame the cause on bad luck, faulty traction, or lack of training and conditioning. Think about how often, especially in the beginning of the season, trainers have to run out on the field to stretch and tend to players who are suddenly downed with muscle cramps and pulls.

Today's star athlete is yesterday's rambunctious kid who engaged in crazy acrobatics in the park. Kids test the limits because they haven't yet defined what the limits are, and often that results in falls and scrapes.

Typically, once they are distressed by the pain of a hard, shocking impact they will weep vigorously and experience the stress response of shaking, similar to the way a dog shakes off water. Shaking or trembling signals that the nervous system is attempting to re-establish body balance. In order to "shake it off," the body must possess a high level of structural stability which in turn yields a high level of elasticity. This shaking lets the brain (specifically the limbic system) understand that danger has passed, thus completing a nervous system response to help release trauma from the body. Once the shock is over, the child will go right back to playing on the same park equipment they were just hurt on. Since most kids exhibit a high degree of flexibility and stability, the next day they typically enjoy the blessing of full pain-free body function.

Although loss of elasticity is an inevitable consequence of advancing age, I am happy to share with you that much of the elasticity we lose can be regained. Optimal muscle tone is solid, yet elastic and relaxed. Defended muscles are more prone to injury and can be overly tight, stiff and painful. Restoration of elasticity does not depend so much on stretching as it does on bringing a new level of structural support to the body and neurologically stimulating defended muscles to regain proper tone. This book will cover how this can be achieved.

The benchmark for superior athleticism has always revolved around strength and power. Although weight lifting builds powerful muscles, there has always been the negative trade off from the consequential body tightness that results from intense muscle training. This extensive increase in muscle tone has been epitomized by the popular term "hard-body." The thing is, to achieve elite status, one must possess not only superior strength, but also the ability to move quickly with precision. That combination allows the athlete to expertly adapt on a moment by moment basis in the ever-changing environment of highly competitive sports.

Stretching Before Activity: Not Always the Answer

Muscle tone is critically important to all movement, even movement that's barely perceptible. Standing still in place requires muscular activity. In order for the body to maintain a completely erect pose, the nervous system must equally and continually activate muscles in the front and back of the body at the same time. Done correctly, the nervous system enjoys a quiet calm from a body successfully able to maintain balance against gravity, in many ways like a precisely. The more highly calibrated the muscle tone, the faster the body can use its proprioceptors, or sensory receptors which cause the body to automatically shift weight and balance.

PNF Stretching Technique

This ability to balance is crucial on the field, and stretching has been shown to increase proprioceptor reaction time. Stretching can also loosen and lengthen muscles and increase flexibility and range of motion. This is why different and innovative ways of direct stretching currently constitute the popular approach to achieve greater levels of elasticity and quickness.

On the surface there is nothing wrong with this. According to the athletic mindset, if you are going to push yourself in the weight room, then push yourself with the same intensity on the stretching mat. However, the problem is that tightness can result from a variety of reasons. If the nervous system is structurally unsteady, whether from prior injury, physical exhaustion, or emotionally on edge, it tightens body muscles to brace itself.

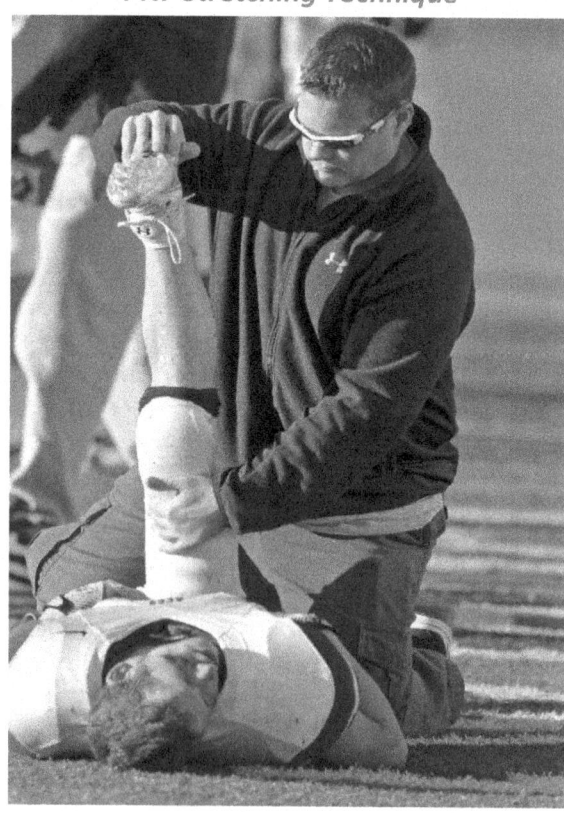

Image 7

A very serious situation takes place in sports when athletes and trainers physically attempt to push through heightened states of physical emergency, known as the FFF defensive reaction.

The resting state of FFF is the mandatory time (even if it's only a split second) when muscle fibers come into neutral and reset for action. This is the safety zone, where the nervous system tells the body an action is completed. If this essential resting state does not happen, muscles become held in FFF defensiveness, as muscle fibers remain on alert.

Forcefully stretching defensive muscles (muscles which have not had a resting state) before action, in order to override the FFF safety mechanism, invites injury. It makes no difference how ingenious the stretching techniques may be. Neurologically speaking, forceful stretching turns off the muscle, handicapping its ability to fire and recoil effectively.

An advanced stretch that overrides the nervous system's muscle control is PNF stretching. Short for proprioceptive neuromuscular facilitation, PNF stretching is done with the assistance of the athletic trainer. Here the athlete severely contracts the muscle by pushing against the trainer's body. When the trainer instructs the athlete to relax, the trainer pushes fairly hard against the hamstring or whatever muscle was previously contracted in order to now stretch it past previous boundaries. (Sharman 2006)

This is an excellent stretch to do *after* a workout or game, but never *before* practice or competition. I am not advocating not loosening up tight muscles before activity. A better approach is walking or doing a slow jog to warm up, then light stretching before engaging in sports.

As stated earlier, there's an issue with many muscle loosening techniques. Intense stretching and even various electrical stimulation modalities can overpower tight muscles and create an illusion of looseness. However, the nervous system will still hold on to the imbalance regardless of muscle flexibility.

The effect of this imbalance is most apparent to the athlete upon awakening the morning after intense physical activity. During the night, the body uses the rest period to reset itself into the old defended pattern which feels safe and ideal to maintain long term survival. Frequently, this reset causes the same muscle to tighten and secure itself just a little tighter than before.

Stop start motions, a feature of most sports, requires an abundance of elasticity within muscle tissue. But the ability to stretch is not, of itself, an indicator of neurological facilitation. Therefore, when resistance has been set in deeply enough or for a long enough time, PNF stretching before practice or competition may no longer be a practical option for relief. Inadvertently, a trainer may be setting a player up for failure on the field in the belief that a stretched muscle is neurologically balanced when in reality it has lost a great deal of its recoil ability.

If you hold a large coil in two hands and stretch it, if there's enough elasticity in it, it will spring back. If there is not enough elasticity, you'll just have a loose coil.

Muscles by their very nature are elastic meaning that they contract and then release to contract again. What distinguishes a good player from a great player is the ability to immediately stop, turn on a dime, and explosively accelerate. The one key ingredient behind all these dynamic feats is elasticity, or the ability to contract and compact the body and dynamically spring forth out of that position.

If massage and other types of bodywork become routine before practice, it's an indication that the nervous system has become too resistant to change. The old pattern has just become too ingrained into the nervous system to be reset by stretches and other means. Adaptation suffers. Once adaptation becomes compromised, performance goes down and injuries go up.

Many athletes today pride themselves on their limberness. However as previously introduced, there is a marked difference between the natural limberness we all experienced during childhood, and what is felt after an intense PNF stretching session.

Think back to your childhood and recall your frustration when the gym teacher forced all the kids to stretch before running. Back then chances are you considered stretching a waste of time. If you wanted to run, you just ran. Your young body was naturally limber and agile. Muscle pulls were almost nonexistent, and you could probably just shake off a twisted ankle or knee injury easily and go right back to the activity that caused you pain. Note that as the years passed, stretching before activity became an ever-greater priority.

Progressive Tightness Affects Athletic Performance

If underlying conditions in the nervous system are not addressed, an athlete's body can move through a progression of levels as depicted by the following chart. These levels can be comparable to a school's grading system. In my experience with patients, an athlete's movement through the levels is not as dependent on age as it is on nervous system resolution. In other words, an older athlete provided with the opportunity to resolve trauma at the deepest level throughout their career will tend to fare far better than others of the same chronological age who are overly burdened with neurological "baggage".

State of the Nervous System and Athletic Performance Observations

"Grade Level"	Description	Observations and Consequences
A	Most often a young athlete	<ul><li>Stable structure and precise muscle firing patterns allow for maximal adaptation</li><li>Can easily take big hits or overly exhaust their body and feel no repercussions</li><li>Nervous system perceives the skeletal structure strong and intact</li><li>Muscles are able to vigorously activate, then properly rest before the next activation</li></ul>

"Grade Level"	Description	Observations and Consequences
B	Hard physical contact, over-exertion or poor nutrition built up over time	• Body muscles are required to remain activated longer then optimal • Tight muscles have created tight protective fascia • Overemphasis on muscle activation is preventing the nervous system from properly rebuilding and maintaining ligaments in a state of high strength and elasticity • Physical feelings of "guarding" or stiffness • Tenderness on application of pressure • Possible reduction in agility
C	Tightness has transitioned to instances of pain	• Reduced agility • Skeletal stability is progressively comprised, and muscles are "on" longer than designed to be • Pain can be lessened by massage and aggressive stretching • Sometimes pain goes away by itself but returns • Nervous system is "robbing Peter to pay Paul" as smaller supportive & finesse muscles are put out of commission in lieu of continually activating the bigger more powerful muscles
D	If still playing, are hurt often	• Inability to turn on a dime or react quickly • Structural instability is significant, along with the continual muscular contractions • Player is continually seeking treatment in the training room getting taped, iced, heat, massage, electrical modalities and anti-pain/inflammation injections • Smaller muscles have atrophied from disuse • Have to retire, are cut, or get replaced at the end of the season
F	Constant pain issues	• Barely any skeletal stability • Continual muscular contractions and cramps • Most likely not active on a team

"The Last Shot": The Importance of Flow

In 1998 the Chicago Bulls faced the formidable Utah Jazz in that year's NBA Finals. Although the Bulls were up three games to two, the momentum had shifted to the Jazz, and the last two games would be played in Utah.

Up to that time few teams had won game seven on the road. To make things worse, Michael Jordan's key support man, Scottie Pippen, was hobbled with a back injury and was only able to contribute 26 minutes. It seemed like everything was against Chicago for that game.

The competition was fierce and with less than one minute in the 4th quarter the score was tied. Suddenly Utah's John Stockton hit a three-pointer which gave the Jazz the lead with just 41.9 seconds left. Completely mentally engaged in the game and with an energized focus, Jordan traveled the length of the court in a mere four seconds to score two points. With the lead cut to just one point, Chicago's defense stepped up, and then Jordan, by immersing his entire being in the present moment, strategically positioned himself in the perfect location to steal the ball from Carl Malone, and score the game-leading bucket. With just 5.2 seconds left, the Jazz tried to launch one last long outside jump shot. With that missed shot, the Bulls won by one point, and Michael Jordan willed his team to another championship. That achievement will forever be remembered as "The Last Shot."

That night Jordan demonstrated how an elite player can transcend circumstances and achieve virtual perfection on the court. This state of physical transcendence is known as "being in the flow" or "in the zone".

The flow state is a paradox where there is tremendous calm amongst dramatic and often violent activity. In this state the mind and nervous system remain calm and centered within a firestorm of outside activities.

In the book *Flow: The Psychology of Optimal Experience,* author Mihaly Csikszentmihalyi quotes Sports Psychologist Dr. Jay Granat as he describes flow as a state of virtual ecstasy often equated with stepping into an altered state of mind. He writes:

> The zone (flow) is a state of mind which is marked by a sense of calmness. In addition, there is a heightened state of awareness and focus. Actions seem effortless and there is an increased belief that your dreams or goals can become achievable and real. In addition, there is also a sense of deep enjoyment when the person is in this unique, special and magical state of being. (Csikszentmihalyi 1990)

Talk to any athlete about being in the flow, and watch their eyes light up with recollections of the intensely memorable instances when they achieved the flow state. This state, by nature, is elusive. In this state intense effort and willpower suddenly transform into calmness and an absolute inner confidence that every action taken will end in triumph. Baseball players in flow report that the ball looks like a slowly pitched grapefruit. Basketball players report that the basket takes on the width of a trash can.

When exceptional training is paired with strong, dexterous, and elastic bodies, then athletes possess the best chance of not only getting into flow but more importantly maintaining that much coveted state.

Accomplished athletes agree that before anyone can experience even fleeting moments of flow, one must put in the time with consistent and focused practice to internalize the necessary routines of their chosen sport. During the random times that flow is achieved, the result is a beautiful synergy of mind and body. Training simply takes over. It's like an auto-pilot switch inside gets triggered. Instead of continually making the split-second decisions competitive action requires, the mind suddenly and simply relaxes. In an instance the athlete moves from an intense active participant to a mentally calm spectator in their own body. While in this deep state of peace, the athlete is fully present literally witnessing their own body performing practiced moves perfectly. This can be described as the moment as when "the dancer becomes the dance."

For athletes who have never experienced flow, the body stabilizing and nervous system rebalancing principles in this book can move the athlete closer to making the flow state a reality. This knowledge is priceless because the better an athlete can assess and maintain flow, the more phenomenal their performance becomes within their chosen field of play. Just as important, many nagging injuries as well as "freak accidents," like hamstring pulls, twisted joints and pulled or ripped ligaments and tendons dramatically decrease.

For non-athletes, these same principles work just as well to re-center and bring a high level of calm to the nervous system. This combination is the magic formula to unlocking tight bodies and relieving chronic pain and painful conditions.

Flow is a Habit

Behind the mystery of this almost mythical state, flow is essentially a deeply ingrained habit within the nerve pathways of the brain and subconscious mind. Remember that Hebb's rule can be summarized as "nerves that fire together, wire together." When a thought or action is continually repeated, those nerves will then fire along the same pathways or synapses. It is this reinforcement which creates a "wiring together" from the standpoint that it takes less and less input or stimulation to fire off and activate a very strong physical, quick and precise response.

In order to achieve flow, the first criteria that must be met is the most obvious. The athlete must practice their moves enough times to both impregnate and integrate the nervous system with a specific and continual pattern of thought coupled with specific action. This nervous system assimilation takes time and concentrated effort. Hall of Fame and legendary football coach Vince Lombardi said it best, "Practice does not make you perfect. Perfect practice makes you perfect."

If an athlete's action and concentration is haphazard and sporadic, then those chaotic patterns are what imprints within the nervous system. In the book *The Power of Habit: Why We Do What We Do in Life & Business*, Charles Duhigg features Hall of Fame football coach Tony Dungy. Coach Dungy took Vince Lombardi's quote to heart by making his playbook simple and basic. Dungy understood that simple plays executed flawlessly yield more success than complicated or flashy trick plays. Although complex plays looked good on the drawing board, by the time the stress and exertion of game time situations wore down the players' abilities to quickly adapt, Dungy knew the only thing he could count on were the core plays he drilled into his players. Simple plays run over and over again in time deeply ingrained themselves into the very fiber of a player's muscle memory. This way, even if playing while hurt, Dungy's players would still execute while the opposition would often falter. (Duhigg 2014)

The second facet for successful achievement of flow is more elusive. It depends expressly on the willingness of the nervous system to let itself go and fully activate its pre-programmed moves without regard to body safety. For the nervous system of an athlete to fully allow the self to be carried by the momentum of flow, a sense of security is required. The body must possess enough stability and balance to feel safe enough to run internal programming, even if it is experiencing pain from trauma or exertion. The athlete must have an inner perception that no matter how intense the competitive action becomes; no significant injury or harm will result.

Knowing the Limits

Competitive sports have never been as intense as they are today. Specialized equipment, unique exercise regimes and superior coaching all figure into a formula for success. Today, top athletes overly exert themselves following scientifically advanced methods which encourage the athlete to keep going to the point of exhaustion.

I am all for pushing yourself past limitations, in order to transform yourself into something greater than you are. However, you must approach the nervous system with respect. To ignore your nervous system's pre-set limitations for safety is a recipe for disaster and future physical or mental sabotage. When the nervous system is pushed into areas it has deemed dangerous for survival, its natural response is the FFF stress reaction. When FFF is activated, the nervous system suddenly tightens muscles deemed necessary for protection. Physiologically, blood moves away from the head and central core and moves out to the arms and legs facilitating those parts with the ability to either run away or fight for survival. Although most people know and refer to this reaction as fight/flight, the very first thing the body does is to freeze, by suddenly tightening all available muscles.

The reason so many top-tier athletes are frequently injured today is because they are playing tight. When their nervous systems are stuck in FFF, their defended minds continually contract muscles in much the same way a cobra constricts before striking. Strong and conditioned muscles naturally hold a tightened tone. However, there is a huge difference between competing when the nervous system is stuck in FFF and muscles are continually engaged, versus when muscles are allowed to rest and reset before the next engagement.

If trainers were able to screen their players and assess which athletes were over their neurological limits, those players could be properly neurologically rebalanced. Once their nervous systems calmed and recalibrated to a greater level of confident tranquility, injuries would dramatically decrease, and their level of play would exponentially improve.

A calm nervous system naturally allows muscles and fascia to gain a higher level of elasticity. With greater elasticity the body can better bend without breaking. When a body perceives greater safety, it has a better chance of moving into flow. When the nervous system is calm and the body is elastic, there exists a general sense of wellness within the nervous system that instills deep confidence that he/she can make a play without getting hurt, or with minimal consequences.

The more stress that is relieved, the better the nervous system works. The better it works, the easier it is to enter and maintain flow.

Modern athletes can come back from the intense punishment of today's contact sports by implementing the guidelines detailed in this book to both deeply de-stress as well as reset their nervous systems.

Chapter 4: Pain is a Memory

The Optimal Nervous System

I am a doctor of function in motion. If something is not in motion, it's not functioning. Getting things to move, and the nervous system to function, is the true key to optimal health.

The nervous system is dynamic. It is always moving and adapting the inside environment to the outside world, seeking its ultimate goal which is balance. When a body is compromised due to pain, different muscles get recruited to assist a weaker area, causing the body to contract.

When pain is experienced, and then resolved, it seems to follow that the issue is solved. But when pain results from chronic states of defensive contraction, those symptoms are not the problem. Thus, the original pain or pain within an associated area along the kinematic chain will undoubtedly return.

The ability of the body to function, not the elimination of pain, determines how much balance and elasticity will return to the body. Balance and elasticity go hand in hand, you can't have one without the other. When you feel pain, it must be dealt with. The restoration of balance and elasticity gives the nervous system a higher level of control, because once this is accomplished, as if by magic, the nervous system is suddenly directing a body that is now more structurally sound. This soundness then resonates throughout the structure resulting in progressively less and less pain.

What if instead of fighting and overwhelming the nervous system we work with it and give it what it wants? It wants balance. Besides the structural balance from strong ligaments, firm stability and proper movement around its center line, the last facet of balance is the muscle contraction itself. After a muscle is activated, it must be neurologically deactivated in order to move into its neutral or resting state. Once a muscle completely rests for a split second, it is ready to fire again.

Stuck in FFF

The refined and specialized human nervous system has a tendency to get stuck in FFF.

Memories of withdrawal muscle recoils and stress reactions, which can include physical, mental/emotional or chemical/dietary stresses become trapped in both muscle and connective tissue. Despite the fact that the tissue may have fully healed from the trauma it sustained, the memory is kept active in the neurological system in the form of tightened muscles suck in a perpetual state of limbo.

By the time the nervous system has reached a point of maximal adaptation for that particular level or event, the nervous system is no longer able to fully reset itself back to its ultimate and highest form of balance.

The technique this book advocates uses the body's own reflexes to help muscles complete these ever-present contraction memories buried in neurological pathways. Once the reflexes safely jar the nervous system into the action of quickly activating these stuck muscles on one side and atrophied muscles on the other side, then the perpetual withdrawal memory causing these muscles to stay in contraction simply fades away.

Every withdrawal reaction that is cleared from the neurological or memory pathway allows the nervous system greater precision and control over the body. In essence, the restoration of higher brain control functions to direct the body to more easily adapt to immediate changes in its environment, versus slow to almost impossible adaptation under defensively locked muscles.

Memory Pathways

Each of us understands the world through the filters of prior experiences. In an airport boarding area, some people are visibly nervous and even scared to board the plane, others are happy and excited. Those who appear nervous or afraid perceive the plane as dangerous. Those showing excitement see the plane as a vehicle of pleasure, taking them on a fun ride to a different destination. These two completely opposite emotional states are based on different ways of experiencing the world. Personal experiences cause memory pathways to be developed in the nervous system.

From personal experience, I was toughened up by surviving "Hell Week" (double football practices under a scorching summer sun) when I was young. Now when it's really hot outside, and people complain about how miserable they are, my mind compares the heat of the present day with what it would be like if I was out practicing in full pads, and I honestly don't feel that hot. The way your brain perceives the information coming in determines your feelings, your outlook, and often your personality.

Human bodies are amazing and the brains and nervous systems that run them are still superior to any computer made to date. But for a minute, picture your body as a machine and your brain and nervous system as a computer. Information comes in as vibrations of light, sound, and feelings through the five senses. Your interpretations of the vibrations based upon previous experiences determine whether your perception is neutral, tolerable, pleasurable or painful.

Since the nervous system is like a computer, its pattern is stimulus-response, stimulus- response. This means that vibrational sensations coming in carry patterns of information which the nervous system first has to interpret, then respond to. Your nervous system's response depends on its current state of structural stability, as well as the level of balance it can continually maintain. The better it does this, the more adaptable you are to change, and the happier the nervous system becomes because it feels safe and assured of survival.

Every cell is connected with every other cell via the integrated communication of the nervous system. It has to be that way in order for the nervous system to adapt and survive the outside environment. The right hand certainly does know what the left hand is doing. When the nervous system is working at optimal efficiency, every part of the body gets blood, nerve, and lifeforce flow equally and continuously.

Psychologically, this creates a very confident personality. In athletics, this combination creates an athlete of the highest caliber.

Cellular Memory

Accepted science teaches us that muscle cells are stabilized and supported by what is called the extracellular matrix (ECM). The main supportive structure for cells in this matrix consists of collagen fascial filaments designed to cradle the cells like a form-fitting pillow of loose cotton or like eggs sitting in a soft foam egg crate. The picture below is the way most biology and anatomy books characterize the structure of the ECM. What looks like tree branches is the illustrator's depiction of the facial supportive weave. The big round ball is the actual cell. This picture demonstrates how the facial weave protects and supports the cell just by gently cushioning it.

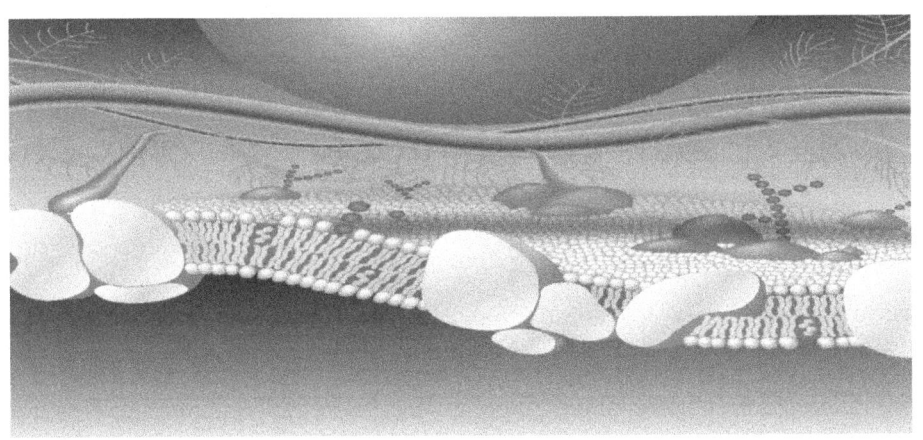

Popular Understanding of the Extracellular Matrix

Image 8

Theory is one thing, but truth can be something entirely different. Extensive research published by Thomas Myers in his book Anatomy Trains paints a different picture from this accepted belief. According to Myers when the nervous system is perpetually caught in a FFF cycle, collagen facial filaments designed to cradle the cell suddenly transform themselves to tension cables which then pull and distort the outer cell wall. (Meyers 2001)

Truer Depiction of Extracellular Matrix

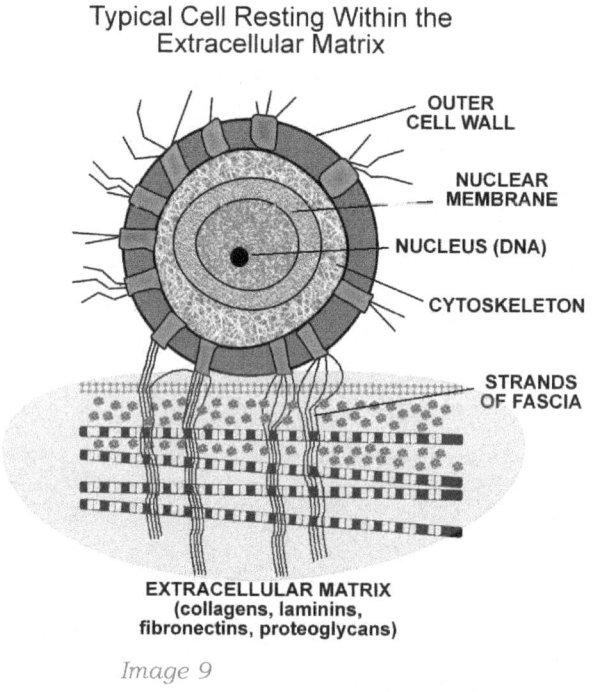

This next picture is a more accurate representation of what actually occurs between the extracellular matrix and each individual cell. Under the constant stress of FFF, muscles and their protective fascial coverings continually tighten. Imagine how those collagen fascial strands, which are supportive in a calm system, will progressively pull against their firm attachment to the outer cell wall when stressed. The harder the pull, the greater the cascade that travels throughout the cell all the way to the centralized DNA.

Typical Cell Resting Within the Extracellular Matrix

- OUTER CELL WALL
- NUCLEAR MEMBRANE
- NUCLEUS (DNA)
- CYTOSKELETON
- STRANDS OF FASCIA

EXTRACELLULAR MATRIX
(collagens, laminins, fibronectins, proteoglycans)

Image 9

This information should act as a wake-up call to all doctors, trainers, chiropractors and body therapists because this increasing pull is a big deal.

When it comes to physiology, Guyton's is the ultimate authority used by all medical schools and other professional colleges who train in healthcare careers. Guyton's will be liberally quoted throughout this book. Guyton's Physiology proclaims that *EVERYTHING IS CONNECTED!*

As stress triggers these fascial filaments to apply continuously heavier and more intense pressure on the outer cell wall, the increased pull deforms the cell. This deformity begins a snowball effect on the inner support structure within the cell itself. Specifically, pull and deformation from the outer cell wall directly causes a microscopic network of protein filaments and tubules called cytoskeleton to pull and deform the cell's nuclear wall. This is a huge deal because inside this wall lies the very essence of what makes up the physical body: the DNA. In the language of cell microbiology, pulls against the cell wall indicate to the body that it is under attack, and must brace itself for survival. Under these conditions the DNA will make subpar proteins, enzymes and other products, because it is working under a state of defense instead of a state of stability and peace.

Scientists validate the above point through current research identifying how stress affects genetic expression. In one study: Genetics of Anxiety and Trauma-Related Disorders by Seth D. Norrholm, PhD, and Kerry J. Ressler, MD, PhD:

> It has become apparent, despite the relatively limited body of literature, that anxiety disorders are the result of multiple, complex interactions between genes and environmental influences.

Several studies on the effect of stress on the DNA expose the dangers of prolonged pressure. In athletics, as well as regular daily life, continual physical stress leads to physical injuries and emotional burdens, reducing one's ability to handle further stress and negatively affecting performance.

Neurological Memory

I'd like to acknowledge someone who has become very influential in my work. Dr. Alan R. Bonebrake has been a mentor who helped me piece together much of the neurology portion of this book.

His genius is in his ability to assemble massive amounts of information from medical and neurological textbooks and apply their core principles and laws in a way that has not been done before. This book has taken those principles and integrated them with information from AK (Applied Kinesiology) and other neurological and chiropractic techniques into a cohesive system of healing. Dr Bonebrake's work is innovative, and you can find more information about his TTAPS technique and training at ttapscenter.com.

Dr. Bonebrake expands on the following Guyton quote: "In contrast to most other sensory receptors pain receptors adapt very little. Pain is basically a *chronic withdrawal reflex* of the brain." (610) (Guyton, Textbook of Medical Physiology, Ninth Edition 1996) According to Dr. Bonebrake, the root cause behind the pain that most people seek care from and medicate against comes from multiple chronic withdrawal reflex reaction memories stuck within the nerve pathways.

Nerve Communication

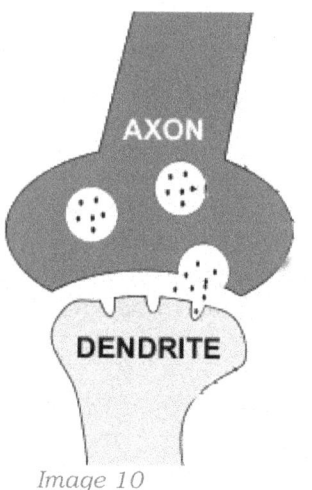

What this means is that the nervous system has held on to the memory of the reflexive movement of the original trauma, or the withdrawal away from pain. So months or even years later, when you move a certain way activating the muscles in the same pattern that you did during the traumatic event, that action will trigger a neurological memory creating muscle contractures that result in physical pain at the site of injury or nearby.

Image 10

Recall the picture earlier in the book of the hand pulling away from the flame. The moment the hand moved, the body formed a neurological memory. The intensity of heat caused momentary trauma which, if prolonged, would threaten survival. This scare cannot be forgotten.

Nerves communicate information by transferring electrical charges from the end of one nerve cell (axon) to the beginning part of another nerve cell (dendrite). This is called the synapses. The signal passes one to the other like old time firefighters, lined up and passing buckets of water to each other. The entire nervous system is a series of connected synapses passing information from one place to another.

Guyton validates this point with the following quote:

> "The storage of information is the process we call ***memory,*** and this, too, is a function of the synapses. That is, each time certain types of sensory signals pass through sequences of synapses, these synapses become more capable of transmitting the same signals the next time, which process is called ***facilitation.*** After the sensory signals have passed through the synapses a large number of times, the synapses become so facilitated that signals generated within the brain itself can also cause transmission of impulses through the same sequences of synapses **even though the sensory input has not been excited.** This gives the person a perception of experiencing the original sensation, although, in effect, **they are only memories of the sensations." (p. 567)** (Guyton, Textbook of Medical Physiology, Ninth Edition 1996)

The explanation above for facilitation explains Hebb's rule, also known as the Law of Facilitation, and most commonly stated as "Nerves that fire together, wire together." The rest of the quote takes you deeper into the Law of Facilitation by validating that the more a certain signal travels through a particular neurological nerve pathway, the more efficient the synapses become at transmitting those pain signals though the entire body. Within a short time, all the brain has to do is think about the pain or previous circumstances creating pain, and that is enough to cause the same quality and intensity of pain as the original event.

The fact that you feel pain indicates that a signal surpassed the established border of safety, commonly called "threshold" in neurology, set up within the nervous system. Once we experience anything (good or bad) the nervous system remembers the combination of signals, as well as the intensity of those signals coming from the five senses, which then create the emotional state. Sensations and emotions result directly from the way individual nervous systems perceive and react to sensory input from the environment.

The more your nervous system experiences the same or similar combinations of sensations the more your nervous system takes after that footpath forming itself into a more open pathway. In time that neurological pathway facilitates so widely that it becomes a virtual road, and as Guyton says, merely thinking/worrying is enough to trigger the same intensity of neurological response of self-protection or pain equal to the original trauma.

Issues in the Tissues: The Second Messenger

In order for the nervous system to maintain parts of the body within a perpetual state of contraction, it institutes a biochemical change inside the cellular structure of the actual nerve cell so that the muscles it controls are able to maintain a continual state of protective contraction. Guyton calls this the "second messenger.

That "second messenger" is the memory of pain held indefinitely within the nervous system.

The second messenger is a major cause of problems as long as it remains active. Every muscle activation which holds second messengers continues to signal the nervous system that something is wrong and/or damaged in that area.

Think of a lion with a thorn stuck in its paw. With every step, he experiences pain. If there is no way he can remove it, his nervous system will adapt by signaling tissues to form a callous in the skin over the thorn. In time, even though he may not consciously feel the intense prick, with every step, his muscles will reflexively contract in order to keep the full brunt of his weight from putting pressure on the affected paw. Certain muscles will begin compensating for others which will tighten connective tissue. His body is establishing the neural pathway discussed in the last section, and this results in one unbalanced lion because now the structure has been affected. That one tiny thorn has now caused the lion to lose dexterity and speed. This puts the lion at a disadvantage in terms of hunting and also at being hunted or having his dominance challenged by a younger loin. Tissue memory of the thorn is the lion's second messenger. The more often second messenger signal patterns present within the nerve cells controlling muscles, the more progressively the muscles tighten over time.

As stated earlier, the nervous system runs on a repetitive pattern of stimulus - response. Sensations enter the brain at varying intensities, on a sliding scale of pleasure on one side, pain on the other. Pleasure causes the nervous system to instinctively open up, pain causes the system to close and protect.

If a muscle contracts, it must receive an "all clear" signal from the nervous system, to allow it to enter a neutral state followed by a repolarization phase where it fully resets for the next firing. It is this "all clear" signal which resolves the second messenger. Sensory fibers are activated when the skin is tapped or swiped, which triggers a muscular reflex within that entire muscle. That reflexive action throughout the muscle is what completes the contraction on one end and the relaxation on the other end, thereby both resetting the tone and clearing the second messenger memory as much as possible.

When the nervous system activates its defensive measures, this memory is long term. In other words, a protectively contracted muscle will remain contracted, because on a deep level the nervous system feels unbalanced, and balance is safety. Safety equals survival. One split second in neutral (an all clear signal) is enough to make neurological changes clearing memory patterns that may have been activating muscle contractures for months, if not years.

In my clinical practice experience, I can verify that these second messengers last for years- and even decades. Once I begin to work with patients stripping away layers of defensive contractions and compensations, it is amazing how memories would suddenly pop into their head about slips, falls and various other accidents they experienced years ago. When I say YEARS, I mean YEARS ago. It is common for a 40+ year old patient to suddenly have a vivid flash of when they fell out of a tree, slipped on the ice, or took a bad hit in competition while in their teens.

When the memory comes, I celebrate that with my patient, because that often means we have stripped away enough compensations to finally arrive at the original event that created the domino effect of problems. The original cause is the weak spot. It is not uncommon to find layers of compensation built over this spot. These layers are the result of additional trauma, over-exhaustion, or muscle activation close to the trauma, when the muscle tightened to defend against another occurrence.

An original cause established in youth is typically below the level of everyday consciousness because the young have a level of elasticity in the tissues which makes it seem all is well. It is only discovered when that site has layers of compensation built up to a point where stiffness or pain results. Pain is a signal that your nervous system has lost the necessary body balance to fully adapt to what you ask your body to do.

Balance and adaptation are not just the key to surviving, they are the key to thriving.

Very often once I balance a patient, they come back complaining of a new pain that "suddenly" showed up, sometimes in a totally different place. After a short time, my patients know me. They feel better when instead of showing concern, I get a big smile on my face and say, "That's awesome!" If a new pain "came out of nowhere", that means the nervous system is feeling strong enough and balanced enough to bring to completion previous muscular traumas it could not properly contract/release. At the time of the original trauma, the nervous system interpreted that its only option was to partially shut down the muscles of the affected area and over activate other muscles, as always, to keep the best balance possible.

Chapter 5: The Vicious Cycle of Pain

Scar Tissue and Microtears

Structures must glide over and through each other; skin over muscles, ligaments and bone; muscles over muscles and bone; nerve trunks and blood vessels through or between muscles and bone; bone over bone; organs over muscles, other organs, peritoneum, and pleura.

Scar tissue inhibits or prohibits this gliding motion, causing relative or complete immobilization, with resulting deconditioning or atrophy, and may compress blood vessels, lymphatic vessels, nerves and other organs, possibly causing obstruction, irritation or inflammation of organ, vessel or nerve function.

Any time a body tissue; such as muscle, tendon, nerves, fascia or ligaments become injured, scar tissue is produced. The extent of injury determines the profoundness of the scar tissue. Even what would seem to be an inconsequential bump may result in microscopic scar tissue being produced as part of the healing process. In ideal situations the body repairs over time. Things like repetitive injury to a certain area, poor nutrition, chronic inflammation, or disease can affect whether or not complete healing can take place.

When the nervous system is forced to live defensively, meaning muscles remain continually tight to brace against attack and maintain skeletal stability, microscopic scar tissue is formed.

Fascia creates the essential elastic weave that holds physical bodies together. The body is designed like a spring to compress, release and reset against multiple forces acting against it. As long as the skeletal structure is strong, and the biomechanical structure is properly balanced against gravity, fascial weaves maintain optimal elasticity. The moment structure and position are compromised by tight muscles following defensive mandates from the nervous system, then all fascial weaves within the compromised area tighten to protect that area. When doctors and trainers treat only the injured area without going deeper into the layers of imbalance, full relaxation is often never achieved because the defensive body is physically unable to regain its optimal neurological neutral resting state.

When fingers are inserted into a Chinese toy, they become trapped. The harder one pulls, the tighter the entire weave compresses, holding the fingers tighter and tighter. The key to escaping this humorous finger trap comes from calming the mind and overriding the nervous system's survival instinct of pulling away. Simply by pushing the fingers in, the entire weave relaxes and expands.

Microscopically, collagen has virtually the same weave pattern as the Chinese finger trap. Similar to the Chinese trap, the more one pulls on fascia (collagen) the more it tightens and constricts. With fascia covering the muscles, the tighter the muscles become as a result of FFF stress, the more the fascia strangles them and tightens the body.

Chinese Finger Trap Toy

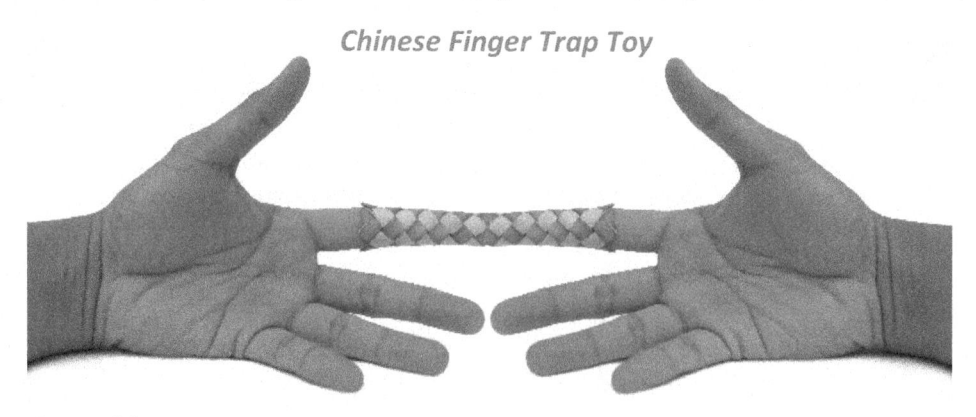

Image 11

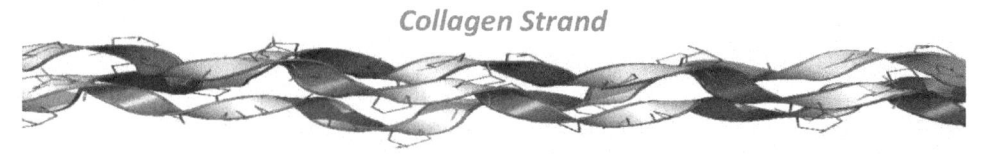

Collagen Strand

Image 12

Lactic acid is the natural biological waste that muscles produce when they contract. Ideally, when muscles relax, the body clears it out. The problem is that acids burn. When the nervous system chronically activates certain muscle groups to defend the body, the buildup of this acid injures and breaks down muscle tissue. Any time tissue breaks down, the injury is considered traumatic, and the body always responds with scar tissue. In the case of a wound, inflammation floods the area with white blood cells to kill pathogens and it lays down scar tissue for stabilization. Likewise, in internal muscle tears, scar tissue is always part of the healing and repair process. There is a difference however, if muscles and body are given a chance to recuperate after scar tissue is formed. When athletes intentionally tear their muscles during workouts, for instance lifting weights, they allow time for the tissues to rest. During the night the body heals the muscles because it is resting in an open posture and the nervous system detects there is no danger that it must defend itself against. Once the area is fully repaired, the scar tissue is naturally disintegrated, and cleared out.

Here's the key point: the healing cycle must be completed neurologically in order for the scar tissue to be cleared out.

Although an area may be medically healed, the memory of the trauma is kept alive and well in the tissues. As long as vulnerable muscles remain stuck within a continuous loop of muscular contractions, those muscles will be continually traumatized, creating varying degrees of pain, soreness and of course, more scar tissue. If the tightness results from muscles held in an overly protective position, as opposed to actual injury, there will be a continual stiffness with pain when attempting to reach or stretch past certain predetermined "safe" boundaries. In many cases where the chief complaint is chronic soreness or pain, the actual cause of discomfort comes from an overactive neurological memory stuck within nervous system pathways keeping that area continually tight, and is not due to tissue damage from the original injury itself. Restoring full elasticity of ligaments, tendons, and fascia may take over a full year to reach optimal function.

Phases of Healing: How Microscopic Scar Tissue Develops

Injured tissue develops microscopic scarring during the early phases of healing. Distinct from the formation of scar tissue, the fibrotic process is the development of fibrous connective tissue. While the scar formation process has a distinct beginning and end, the fibrotic process will continue forming in tissue as long as an irritant exists.

According to Bonica's Management of Pain (Third Edition) there are three phases of healing. These phases are described as follows:

Three Phases of Healing

PHASE	KNOWN AS	TIME LENGTH	CHARACTERISTICS	BODY RESPONSE
1	Acute Inflammatory Phase or Reaction Phase	Up to 72 hours	Inflammation Bleeding Edema Swelling Redness Acute Pain	Release of antibacterial anti-inflammatory enzymes to break down damaged tissues (histamines serotonin prostaglandins).
2	Repair Phase or Regeneration Phase	48 hours to 6 weeks	Low oxygen tension. Hypoxia from edema. Loss of flexibility and range of motion.	Above substances released, plus the addition of phagocytes to remove cellular debris. Collagen fibers are disorganized at this point.

3	Remodeling Phase	3 weeks to 12+ months	Improved tensile strength of the tissues. Controlled exercises required.	Remodeling of collagen in tendons and ligaments. Higher level of organization of collagen fibers plus appropriate orientation

These phases are common to all healing, no matter the extent or source of the injury. This means that any physical trauma, from stubbing your toe to open heart surgery must pass through these steps in order for tissue to become whole again. (John D. Loeser 2000)

According to Dr. Bonebrake, some scar tissue is the result of microtears within the muscle and can be caused by either trauma or joint immobilization which leads to tissue deterioration. In time scar tissue dehydrates and shrinks causing further immobilization and further inflammation. For the purposes of this book please note that I'm referring to microscopic scar tissue in muscle and fascia that affects movement, and not scar tissue that naturally results from exercise and weight training.

As a response to injury, collagen appears like a tangled mass of fibers at the microscopic level, not unlike randomly scattered hay. In order to realize full healing these fibers must come into ordered alignment, like a braided rope, so the body can regain the flexibility that collagen affords the tissue. A young body or one devoid of prior injury or layers of compensation, once brought into neurological and physical balance, can achieve this quickly. But typically, neurological needs- specifically completion of the activation/relaxation cycle and the resetting of the muscles for firing- is not addressed at the time of injury. If left unaddressed, inability to complete the neurological cycle promotes further damage and, over time, pain increases.

Small Muscle Atrophy

By continually tightening certain muscle groups, other smaller muscles transition into disuse and atrophy. Usually these smaller muscles are close to the spine or right next to movable support joints like ankles and knees. They act as stabilizers and as the critical starters of motion.

Think of these muscles as the first gear on a stick shift car. First gear is designed to start the car's motion. Once past 10 MPH, the driver shifts into second gear. As long as the road is flat, a car can be started in second gear, but it's a choppy and awkward start. This is what happens once the nervous system gets locked into a pattern of continual defense and the body gets tighter, where a common practice employed is stretching to loosen muscles. However, this begins another repetitive cycle, producing

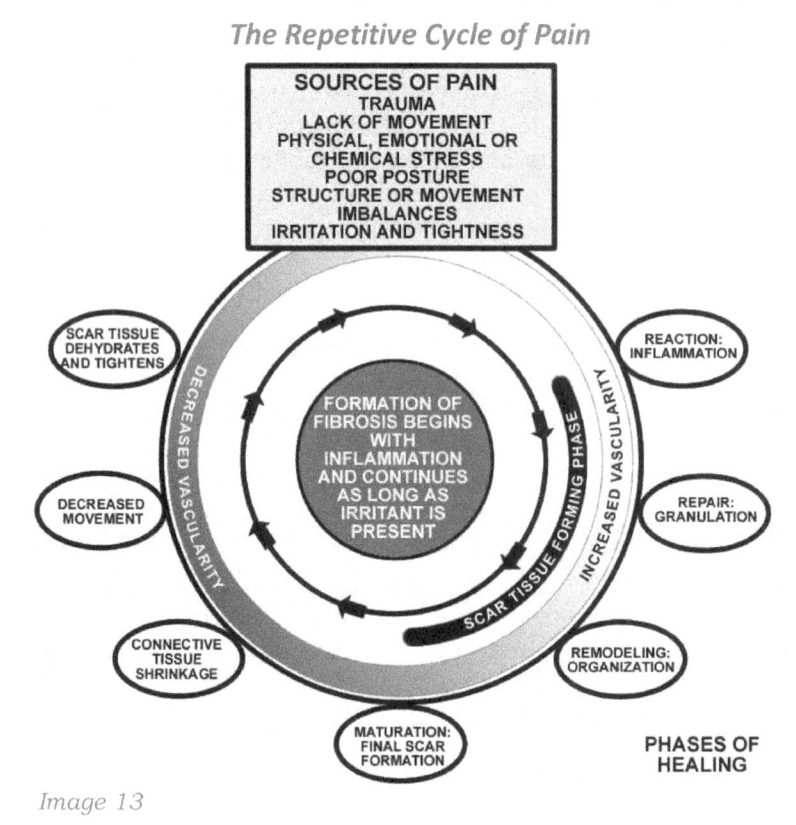

The Repetitive Cycle of Pain

Image 13

increasing degrees of imbalance and muscle tightness. As larger muscles tighten, small supportive muscles atrophy.

With more physical exertion comes greater imbalance. This is what I see and help to resolve daily in clinical practice through functional testing and evaluation of the nervous system. The energy necessary to run a physical body will flow appropriately or it will get locked and trapped. If a practitioner can keep the energy flowing and the body stable yet moving freely, an athlete (or chronic pain patient) can maintain a higher level of adaptability, which brings with it the fringe benefit of pain free muscles.

The Pain Cycle

We have discussed numerous sources of pain so far. Each of these will follow the same progression through affected body tissues. The first phase of repair features inflammation. Throughout the course of this intense healing phase, vascularity is increased in order to bring oxygen, repair chemicals, and other components to the cells while removing pathogens and cellular debris. Newly synthesized collagen is then laid down, initially haphazardly, and then in a more organized way. The completion of scar tissue formation signals the end of the healing phase. Here, scar tissue will respond to manual therapy.

Remember the earlier section about the second messenger and the example of the lion with the thorn in his paw. The presence of the second messenger can keep the muscles held tightly. The problem is that muscles can only stay contracted for a short time before the buildup of lactic acid breaks down muscle tissue, causing greater levels of inflammation. Acid is one of three ways to break down or denature protein, the other two being salt and heat. Muscles are made of protein. Lactic acid causes muscle scar tissue, through this denaturing process.

Now, or at any time after this phase, once body tissue is satisfied with neurological completion, microscopic scar tissue will be naturally absorbed into the system. *But until tissue can be neurologically satisfied it remains in FFF. Tissue in FFF is subject to pain and an ongoing pain cycle.* (Cantu and Grodin 1992)

Any time microscopic scar tissue is present, it's a sign that the healing process was short-circuited. So, although qualified medical professionals or objective tests may determine a wound or trauma has been completely healed, that hidden scar tissue will act as a perpetual trigger causing the nervous system to continually activate the muscles within the immediate area. The concept of microscopic scar tissue may seem bizarre. However, this is my first suspicion when a patient complains of a "little deep knot," "a constant pain," or something that "just doesn't feel right."

In clinical practice, once my patients are stabilized, properly adjusted, and their muscles neurologically re-engaged, the last thing I look for and clear is this microscopic scar tissue. The very presence of this scar tissue is the reason why patients jump from practitioner to practitioner, doctor to doctor. Many patients become frustrated because, although their sharp and immediate pain from an injury is gone, residual tightness, soreness or nagging aches remain. From experience, I can safely say the pain or discomfort will unfortunately remain until the affected muscle is neurologically commanded to complete its contraction and enter its neutral state whereby the activation/relaxation cycle is resolved. Only then does the patient feel the freedom of movement without any catch or pain.

Layered Compensations

Note that in the chart we discussed in the last section, the cycle of pain progresses beyond the maturation phase when the final scar tissue is formed. If there is a need for immobilization, because of pain for example, connective tissues may shrink. In addition, when collagen is initially laid down in a haphazard way during the initial healing phase, it can decrease tissue extensibility. The dehydration of scar tissue is another factor that inhibits movement. Scarring is non-vascular, so the more scar tissue that was developed during the healing, the less blood and lymph can circulate in the affected area.

If you look at the top of that image, you can clearly see that several of the points just mentioned are causes of pain, causing the cycle to repeat itself. The more immobility, the more tissue breakdown results, which is followed by inflammation, followed by scar tissue, and so on.

Although an area may be medically healed, the memory of the trauma is kept alive and well in the tissues. As long as vulnerable muscles remain stuck in a continuous loop of muscular contractions, those muscles will be continually traumatized, creating varying degrees of pain, soreness and of course, scar tissue. If the tightness is the result of muscles held in an overly protective position, as opposed to actual injury, there will be continual stiffness with pain when attempting to reach or stretch past certain predetermined "safe" boundaries. In many cases where the chief complaint is chronic soreness or pain, the actual cause of discomfort comes from an overactive neurological memory stuck within the nervous system pathways keeping that area continually tight, and not from the original injury.

An unbalanced nervous system, left on its own, will suffer from compromised structural stability, which unfortunately grows progressively weaker. The unbalanced patient is doomed to a continual cascade of muscular contractions along with an increase in muscular atrophy. The ensuing pain occurs from tight muscles and constricted fascia strangling the ability to move freely, or from weak muscles unable to properly maintain a contracted state during specific body postures or movements.

At some point during the pain cycle, the nervous system will find its "best balance possible at that time" in accordance with whatever compensations need to be made. These compensations can include long term recruitment of muscles into work they were never intended to do. Once the best balance possible is achieved, a layer of compensation is established. But remember, "best balance possible" is not ideal. If scar tissue remains, if the second messenger is not satisfied, or if the area is again traumatized, the cycle begins anew. Once again, the cycle begins and inflammation leads to additional microtears which promote additional scar tissue. At this point a new "best balance possible" needs to be found along with additional muscle compensation. This is the formation of an additional layer of compensation.

These compensations build up in layers over one another. Over time, the pain becomes greater and involves more body tissue. The muscles become ever tighter due to increased nerve pulsations. Every layer the nervous system is forced to take on sacrifices efficiency for safety, and the end result is poor neurological muscle tone and a compromised ability to adapt. So, in treatment, each layer which is stripped away improves tone and increases adaptability.

Jenga Puzzle

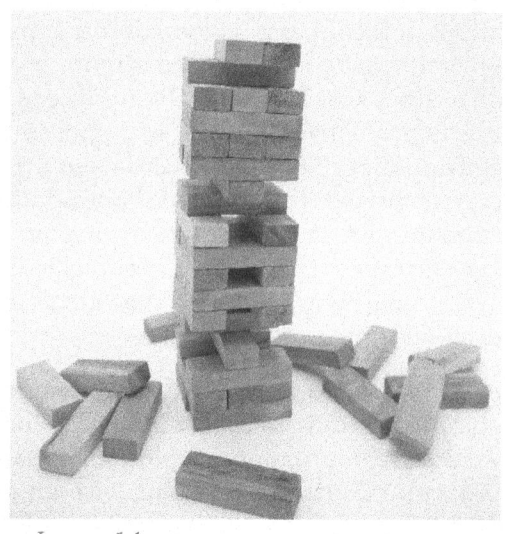

Image 14

To clarify layering, think about a Jenga puzzle. To play the game, participants take turns pulling blocks out of a somewhat dubiously balanced stack. With each piece removed, the puzzle becomes more structurally unstable.

This instability can be compared to a body whose ligaments have lost structural integrity. Once ligaments are unable to hold the body in balance against gravity, muscles are recruited for this task. In the picture, you can liken the blocks lying beside the puzzle to muscles which simply were unable to compensate any longer for ligamental laxity. These are the muscles which, over time, have become "turned off," atrophied, or held hostage by fascia, thus rendering them useless for balance. As the nervous system deems these muscles ill equipped for the task, additional muscles are employed in order to hold the best balance possible. These muscles are tasked to work overtime to continually compensate for this ongoing imbalance, and, over time, physical structure becomes increasingly unsteady and it leans.

During treatment, each revitalized muscle constitutes a balance point, tantamount to putting one more block back into the puzzle structure. With each piece replaced, or each muscle turned back on, greater structural integrity is achieved. As structural strength improves, the nervous system feels safe to relax and reorient tight muscles out of their perpetual "death-grip" status, and closer to their ideal tone. Ideal tone is characterized by the nervous system's ability to precisely turn muscles on and off, and to keep just the right amount of muscular contraction to hold the body upright and mobile, without the extremes of any long term overly contracted muscles.

Chapter 6: Reflexes Are More than a Tap on the Knee

Resetting the Nervous System

Experiencing the pain of fire causes an almost instantaneous flexion of a hand away from the flame. But that's only half the story. What happens is that as the arm flexes, the opposite side of the body extends away from the source of the threat. So, if you touched the flame with your right hand, your right hand and arm would flex up, and simultaneously the muscles on the left side of your back would contract into extension, pulling your entire body away. Combined, the entire reaction is called a flexion/extension withdrawal reflex, or a crossed extensor reflex.

The flexion/extension withdrawal reflex happens when two or more muscles are forced by the nervous system to recoil away from something it perceives as dangerous. When this happens, one muscle may become stuck in an active firing position while its opposite muscle is stuck in an inhibited or deactivated state.

The true key for resetting the nervous system is completing both the firing process as well as the deactivation that results from an incomplete flexion/extension withdrawal reflex.

As you will see later in this chapter, stimulating reflexes can be used to complete neurological cycles which have led the nervous system to tighten tissues.

Injuries in sports, as well as in daily life, will always happen. Bodies are not indestructible. However, if this information about the way the nervous system truly works is accepted and acted upon, it is my sincere hope that devastating injuries from muscle over-use will dramatically decrease. Instead of coaches, trainers and fans ascribing sports injuries to bad luck or poor training, we can treat at the root cause: the overwhelmed and overprotected nervous system. Medical and structural specialists can stop blaming instability merely on "old age".

The Nervous System as a Computer

In order to understand how a nervous system can be calmed, you must first understand what the nervous system is and how it can safely be controlled. Broken down to its bare essentials the nervous system is like a computer. Computers work on the simple premise of stimulus-response-stimulus-response. That means the type of command entered produces a direct programmed response. A different command will achieve a different response.

Stimuli creating neurological responses take the form of vibrations. Eyes respond to light vibrations creating images in the brain which we call sight. Sound vibrations cause the inner ear to vibrate creating for us the sense of hearing. Touch is merely the stimulation of sensing receptors within the skin which transmit signals to the brain for interpretation. Depending on the intensity of the energetic signals, brains either judge them as pleasurable and life-giving or painful and threatening. The point is that stimuli into the nervous system comes in as vibrations, creating appropriate reflexive preprogrammed responses. Depending on the current level of stability, safety and balance, your nervous system can and will tolerate different levels of vibrational intensity. If your skin can tolerate heat, then the warmth of summer sun will be perceived with pleasure. However, once you get sunburned, the same intensity of sun will now newly register as pain.

Responses to vibrational stimuli from the sense organs occur as preprogramed reflexes. It is important to understand that last sentence, because it sets the foundation for the practitioner to actually manipulate the nervous system.

Reflexes and Sense Receptors

The following Guyton's quote validates that the nervous system responds to vibrational stimulation from the sense organs with reflexive responses, which are then transmitted to ALL parts of the body. Think differently from what has been popularly taught and assumed about the body: a headache has nothing to do with knee pain, or a sore ankle has nothing to do with a sore wrist, because they are in different parts of the body. Read for yourself what the ultimate authority in medical science says about how intimately the body is connected:

From Guyton's 9th Edition:

> ...**sensory information from the receptors of the entire body surface** and from some deep structures...enters the central nervous system through the peripheral nerves and is conducted to multiple sensory areas...signals are then relayed to essentially all other parts of the nervous system... (pp. 566-567) (Guyton, Textbook of Medical Physiology, Ninth Edition 1996)

Let's break down the quote and look at it in greater detail. "**Sensory information from the receptors of the entire body surface**," speaks volumes for how the nervous system keeps tight control of the body, and more importantly what we can do to manipulate it later on. The "sensors" Guyton's discusses are the billions of neurological sensory cells abundant within every inch of skin from surface to deep layer, and even in soft tissue. For the purposes of this book we will concentrate mainly on skin and connective tissue (ligament and tendon) sensors.

Now take a look at the rest of that quote:

> "...enters the central nervous system through the peripheral nerves and is conducted to multiple sensory areas...signals are then relayed to essentially all other parts of the nervous system..."

What "enters" into the central nervous system through the peripheral nerves (nerves from outside into center) are informational signals which are then relayed to all other parts of the nervous system all the way to the cellular level. Every signal that enters into the body is almost instantly communicated throughout the system to every other part of the body. This communication has to be this way in order for the brain to keep tight control over all body movements, especially gait. Gait is the individualized rhythmic pattern of a person's walk.

Imagine while walking along a sidewalk you suddenly bump your shoulder on the corner of a wall. At impact, every part of the body is immediately aware of the collision. Within a split second, your nervous system makes the exact muscle contraction calculations necessary to the pull away from the wall. Once out of harm's way, the nervous system, if able, will once again regain both its bearings and its balance. You will continue walking, this time being a little more careful not to hit your shoulder again.

Guyton confirms the stimulus-reflexive response, stimulus-reflexive response computer design of the nervous system by adding:

> "The major function of the nervous system is to process incoming information in such a way that appropriate motor responses occur."

Now that we have established the exacting dominance of the nervous system, a closer look must be taken at the actual sense receptors which are tightly packed and cover every millimeter of skin. Although the mechanoreceptor sensors registering balance changes within joints and ligaments are important, the receptors within the skin play an even more vital role in how the nervous system can be manipulated and reset.

According to Hilton's law, the nerves controlling the joint and its surrounding structures also control the skin over the joint. So, touching the skin, according to this neurological law, has an effect over the structure and movement potential of the joint itself. The important thing to understand here is that skin receptors notify the brain of rates of change within the joint. So, if a neurological cycle can be brought to completion in this way the brain is no longer tasked with retention of the pain memory.

The Role of Nerve Cell Receptors

There are several types of nerve cell receptors which cover the outer skin and are tightly packed within its various levels and layers. For the purpose of simplicity, we will focus on the Ruffini and Pacinian corpuscles (AKA nerve endings). Ruffini corpuscles sense touch, pressure and vibration. They are the ones that register stretches in the skin. Pacinian corpuscles sense higher vibrational frequencies and transient pressures. Here, transient pressures mean sudden changes of pressure against the skin.

Ruffini and Pacinian corpuscles (nerve endings) in the skin look like those little balls given to anxious people to squeeze in order to reduce stress. This unique shape is not accidental. Anatomists know that, within the body, shape determines function. The inner rubber matrix of a stress ball allows it to recoil back to its original shape once outer pressure is released.

From a practical standpoint, remember everything picked up by our five senses is vibrational in nature. These vibrations come in different frequencies so we are able to sense the differences between a soft sound and a loud noise or the sensations of a feather traveling across your skin, and a slap. They are all vibrations, one less intense, while another is more powerful.

What you hear, feel, taste, smell and see is not so much dependent on the vibrational stimulus coming in as much as the quality of the signal the sense organ transmits to the brain.

In early artillery wars, many soldiers who fired cannons did not wear ear protection. The continual high vibration jolts to the eardrums damaged the ability for the ears to

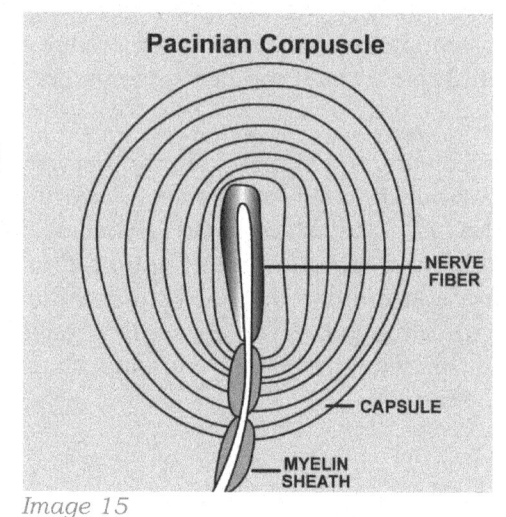

Image 15

register correct sound levels to the brain. Cooks can desensitize their fingers to the point where, as long and they are fast, they can pull out items from boiling water without getting burned. When working with a patient who has layered defensive responses that cause pain, a light touch can register to their nervous system as sharp, stabbing pain. In all these different scenarios, the quality of the signal being transmitted to the brain has been compromised.

Revisiting Hebb's rule, "Nerves that fire together wire together" shows us that in each of these examples a neurological pathway has been established and reinforced by repetition to such an extent that information transmitted has been altered.

Ion Channels & The Sodium- Potassium Pump

Recall that Ruffini and Pacinian corpuscles are shaped like balls. Sense receptors communicate specific signals to the brain based upon which particular corpuscle gets squeezed or deformed and where they are located. These sense organs trigger the moment the suddenly deformed outer wall makes contact with the activation tip of the sensory neuron in the cell.

The Ion Channel

Let's keep this simple, this is not a book about physiology, it is a practical book on how to make actual and immediate changes to the body. The sodium potassium pump provides the means for us to feel sensations on the skin, even those as subtle as the touch of a cobweb. It is also the mechanism responsible for muscle activation or firing. When the pressure of a heavy or light touch is applied to ball-shaped sensory neurons (corpuscles), these receptors communicate specific signals to the

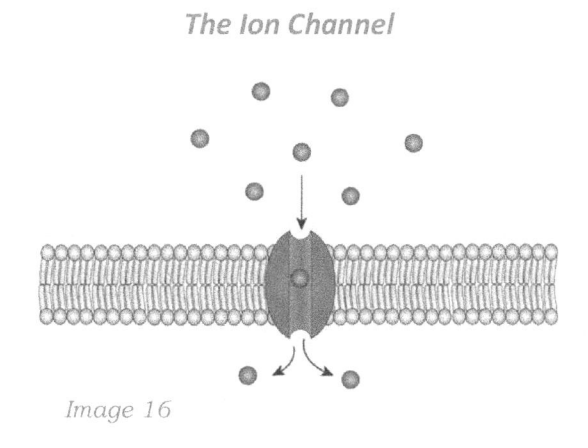

Image 16

brain based upon which particular corpuscles gets squeezed or slightly deformed and where they are located. In practice, the practitioner can release a powerful neurological wave response through a simple light sweep over the skin.

When I treat patients, quick and light therapeutic pressure is applied to the skin in areas where layered defensive responses are present. Recall the last chapter when the second messenger was discussed, this is what I'm referring to here. The second messenger is a memory pattern stuck in a portion of the nervous system track causing continual contraction in muscles.

The neurological wave is released through the sudden deformation that the outer wall of the corpuscle sustains through touch. When deformed, the outer wall actually presses down on the inner activation tip, which then sends an energetic message via nerve cells into not only the skin layers but more importantly the underlying muscle.

When a sensory nerve/corpuscle cell is at rest, there exists an unequal balance of more sodium (Na+) ions on the outside of the cell wall with more potassium (K+) ions within the cell. When in a neutral phase, the membrane of the nerve cell wall connected to the sensory corpuscle (squeeze ball) remains in what is called the resting membrane potential. The moment a touch deforms the squeeze ball it triggers a reaction scientifically known as is depolarization. Here specific border gates along

Nerve Cell (Neuronal Anatomy)

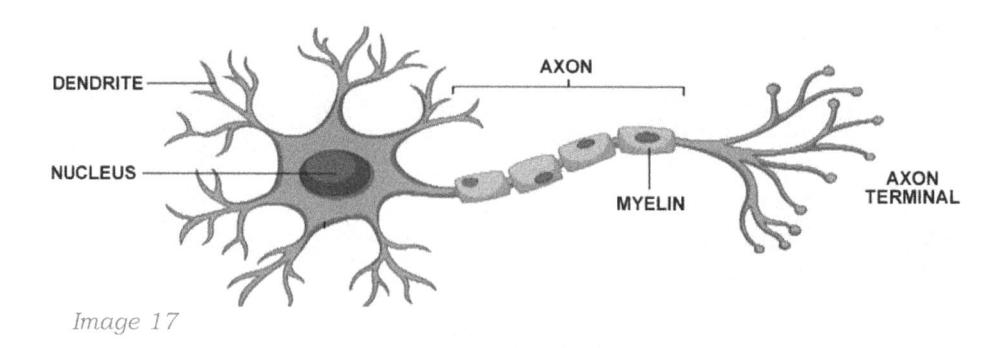

Image 17

Chapter 6: Reflexes Are More than a Tap on the Knee

the outer cell wall of the attached nerve cell called ion channels suddenly open allowing sodium (Na+) ions on the outside to rush in making the inner part of the cell more positive.

The precise chemistry of this is not as important to understand as much as it is to grasp the concept of what actually occurred the moment the sensory squeeze ball deformed when touched. Think of the sparks that jump out the moment two flint stones are suddenly swatted together. The same thing happens inside the neuron or nerve cell connected to the sensory corpuscle. At this depolarization the nerve cell suddenly awakens and it transmits the signal to the next nerve cell in the chain until the signal reaches the muscle causing contraction.

Since the nervous system is all about balance, soon after the original cell fires and sends its signal to the next cell in the chain, the now electrically spent first neuron must go back into a resting state in order to accept future stimulus and to again fire an electrical chemical message. In order

The Sodium Potassium Pump

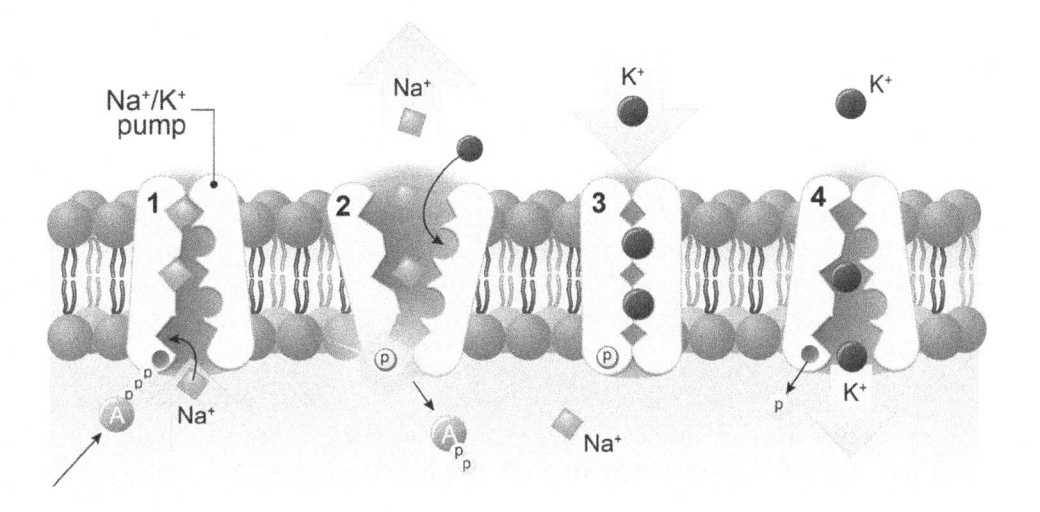

Image 18

for the original cell to rest and recharge it has to actively pump out the inner sodium (Na+) ions that rushed in and pump back in the potassium (K+) ions that escaped. That pumping mechanism is called the sodium/potassium pump. Once balance is restored, the cell is now considered repolarized and the electrical potential along the outer cell wall is restored to the original "resting membrane potential."

At issue here is not the electrical stability at the cell membrane but rather the lack of full and complete relaxation present within the entirety of the muscles the nervous system activated to hold the best position possible during whatever FFF challenge it faced.

This activation principle is called the "all-or-none law." Defined, it states that the *strength of a nerve cell or muscle fiber's response to a stimulus is independent of the strength of the stimulus.* As long as the stimulus exceeds threshold, the nerve or fiber completely activates. So any touch on a sense organ which is stronger than a fly walking across the skin but less harsh than a strong slap, is enough pressure and fits within the safe range to trigger the nerve to fire a reflexive response. Although this last point may seem confusing, think of the last time a medical doctor tapped your knee to get your leg to kick slightly. Called the patellar tendon knee reflex, the rubber hammer hit your knee harder than a touch, but softer than a firm whack. As long as the stimulus was strong enough for the nervous system to feel the blow, but not intense enough to cause discomfort, it reached a safe neurological threshold to activate the reflex.

The "all-or-none law" teaches us that all nerve impulses at threshold fire at either full capacity or they don't fire at all. So, if a muscle fires and then goes into relaxation, how could part of it be stuck in a chronic state of partial contraction while its direct opposing muscle is stuck in a continual deactivation?

The answer lies in neurological tone. Remember that Guyton's stated that the optimal muscle tone is at 1 Hz, and at 1 Hz, the nervous system has achieved its ideal sympathetic resting tone. Through this high level of balance, the nervous system can readily speed up or slow down the system at will. Think of your own car, if it is a few years old, the engine may not be as smooth as it was when you first bought it, but it is still reliable. When parts are older and the engine is not tuned up, you can take a ten-hour trip, but the engine will work harder, the ride will be slightly rougher and you will spend more money on gas. The same thing holds true with your nervous system. When it is stuck in various degrees of FFF, it is working and running harder than ideal. Your body will be tighter and the way it uses energy will be compromised. You may be OK to walk a mile but to run it would wind you badly, and force you to walk towards the end. As your body and nervous system get stronger, jogging a mile is easy and five or ten miles becomes your new challenge. As your nervous system becomes more efficient, your nervous system tone moves ever closer to stabilizing at its ideal balance point.

Please note that when discussing nerve firing, there is a distinct difference between firing *ability* ("all or none") and firing *efficiency* (nervous system tone).

The Nervous System and Reflexes

The most important thing to the nervous system is balance. Balance is survival. Survival is life. At its very foundation, the greater balance the nervous system maintains, the calmer it becomes and the better it works. The secret to getting and staying in athletic flow, as well as attaining exceptional health, comes down to this elementary premise.

When the nervous system is over stimulated and stuck in FFF it causes the body to become tighter due to the dysfunction of both the nervous system and body muscular tone continually moving ever farther away from optimal. The longer the nervous system stays in FFF, the more it must continually compensate. For every stressful imbalance in whatever form it comes, the brain must shift, move and hold the body in the best compensated position possible. Another stress, another shift, another move equates to a tighter hold. As stress builds upon stress these compensations layer themselves in the tissues like an onion.

Remember that, when already in FFF, shocks past a certain predetermined safety range reflexively drive the nervous system more deeply in FFF. This safety range changes over time, becoming a narrower window. Recall Hebb's rule (nerves that fire together wire together), it doesn't take much time or shock to establish a new neural pathway which will reinforce greater levels of danger creating ever tighter muscle patterns.

Once I truly understood the dynamic nature of the nervous system, I began to think that current methods for treating pain and lack of mobility were short-sighted and somewhat superficial in nature. Note, I am not saying ineffective. What I am saying is that relieving pain should not be considered an end goal. Instead, restoring function to the nervous system should be looked upon as a first step for not only rehabilitation but to achieve maximal physical efficiency. To be fair, up until now, there was not much that could be done to functionally strip away compensatory layers and rebalance the nervous system for more long-term effectiveness.

The bulk of information on how to reset the nervous system comes from the brilliant observations of established scientists, doctors and neurologists who presented and documented their findings in classically accepted core medical and neurological textbooks.

Because he helped me reach a deep understanding of these great thinkers, I am most indebted to the research of my mentor Dr. Alan R. Bonebrake. It was through his research that I was able to provide you with all these pertinent points from Guyton's Physiology. In studying body reflexes, Dr. Bonebrake states that his break-through came when he concluded that if reflexes have been used for years to *diagnose* areas of neurological dysfunction, then why couldn't these same reflexes be used to *treat* those very dysfunctions?

A reflex reaction results when nerve stimulation directly causes a specific and dynamic muscle activation with a precise part of the body. Typically, this can happen naturally to move the body away from danger, for example when moving a hand away from a flame. Physicians use reflexes as an assessment tool. By stimulating the nerve cells during a neurological exam, they gain an understanding of the presence as well as the strength of different reflexes. Deep tendon reflexes are responses to muscle stretch. One example of this reflex is the knee-jerk experienced when the physician uses a small hammer to tap the patient's leg. This particular reflex test is used to assess the integrity of the spinal cord in the lower back.

Utilizing what Dr. Bonebrake teaches in his marvelous TTAPS course, I was able to purposefully use specific reflexes to manipulate the nervous system to fully activate and restore more optimal tone. The more optimal the tone the more calm, efficient and pain free the body becomes.

Tight muscles and structurally unsound postures are the nervous system's attempt to balance itself, but these cause chronic pain. Specific stretching, tetanizing electrical current or other rigorous modalities can be used to exhaust and relax muscles. But the moment the nervous system gets a chance to reorder and reorganize itself, it will revert back to the disordered pattern.

A reflex can be used therapeutically to instantaneously open up the nervous system to accept change. The reflex allows the nervous system to reset itself, and as long as that change is reinforced, long term changes will occur.

Understanding Reflex Reactions

Once I understood these reactions, I was able to comprehend the elegance as well as the power behind what is required to make significant functional changes to the nervous system.

Three points are valuable to remember when understanding reflex reactions. First, the nervous system is like a computer that runs the body. It works on a moment by moment, stimulus-response, stimulus-response basis. It has no sense of time - there was no yesterday, and there is no tomorrow. There is only the ever-present NOW. Right at this moment, the only thing on its agenda is to keep the best balance possible. The better it keeps everything organized and within established parameters, the better it can effectively command inner metabolism and outer musculature to adapt to the ever-changing environment.

Second, adaptation is characterized by the nervous system's ability to complete a current cycle of activity and quickly initiate a new and more appropriate cycle. Whether employing the sympathetic or parasympathetic nervous system, this function's goal is again, to reach balance.

Third, although every stimulus challenges the current state of balance, the manner and degree of reflexive response is determined by *the total amount of defensive load being born by the nervous system*. Most people are burdened with multiple layers of re-alignments and compensations, like an onion in tiered levels, over the course of months and years. The younger the person, the more punishment and compensations their body can handle without conscious awareness of anything wrong.

In order to know how to placate the nervous system and resolve layers of compensation and resistance, an understanding of reflex reactions is important. There are two types of reflex reactions. The one known as the positive stretch reflex is defensive, as it locks up muscles or muscle groups and surrounding fascia. The negative stretch reflex is equalizing, and designed to keep tight control over the nervous system.

Let's look more deeply at positive and negative stretch reflexes.

The Positive Stretch Reflex

When discussing the positive stretch reflex, remember how muscles activate. Direct pressure, movement or vibration on sensory nerve corpuscle cells (the squeeze ball-like structures) deforms their shape, causing depolarization. In addition, it stretches little spring-like mechanisms within the muscles called the spindle cells. These spindle cells cause the muscle activation.

> "The simplest manifestation of muscle spindle function is the muscle stretch reflex (also called myotatic reflex [muscle spindle stretch reflex] – that is, whenever a muscle is stretched, excitation of the spindles causes reflex

contraction of the large skeletal muscle fibers of the same muscle and closely allied synergistic muscles...

"The stretch reflex can be divided into two components...the dynamic stretch reflex is elicited by the potent dynamic signal transmitted from the primary endings of the muscle spindles, caused by rapid stretch of the muscle. That is, when a muscle is suddenly stretched, a strong signal is transmitted to the spinal cord, and this causes an instantaneous strong reflex contraction of the same muscle from which the signal originated thus, *the reflex functions to oppose sudden changes in the length of the muscle because the muscle contraction opposes the stretch...* (p.689) (Guyton, Textbook of Medical Physiology, Ninth Edition 1996)

As you read Guyton's description of the positive stretch reflex, note the part where it says:

Excitation of the spindle cells causes reflex contraction of the large skeletal muscle fibers of the same muscles and closely allied synergistic muscles.

Now note how in the second section it says after a sudden stretch, an instantaneous strong reflex contraction takes place within the same muscles where the signal originated from. This positive reflex is designed for protective measures. It bears down, making sure that no more trauma happens to that area. Here is the problem, the last bit of the quote says:

The reflex functions to oppose sudden changes in the length of the muscle because the muscle contraction opposes the stretch....

That last part explains how this protective reflex could be your worst enemy. What is supposed to be a caretaker winds up being your jailer. According to Hebb's rule, when something goes wrong in the nervous system it tends to stay wrong.

Once the positive reflex locks up a muscle, not only is that muscle affected, but other nearby muscles which act to assist in similar tasks become activated to re-enforce muscular contractions in the area which has been deemed vulnerable by the nervous system. For example, the rectus femoris is responsible for lifting the leg. When stuck in a defensive mode, the nervous system will feel forced to recruit and also overly tighten the vastus lateralis, the vastus medialis, the sartorius, and the iliopsoas to perform this task. The net result is cramps or overly constricted front leg muscles.

In essence, the positive stretch reflex brings with it a snowball effect. Once it starts, if unchecked, impairment becomes progressively worse as additional areas of the body tighten.

The Negative Stretch Reflex

The negative stretch reflex is a function of the part of the nervous system that promotes homeostasis (optimal balance). This particular aspect, called the parasympathetic nervous system, is responsible for triggering activity for such diverse functions as regulating temperature, and proper digestion. Note Sherrington's Law:

> When a muscle is **suddenly shortened**, exactly opposite effects occur because of decreased nerve impulses from the spindles. If the muscle is already taut, any sudden release of the load on the muscle that allows it to shorten will elicit both dynamic and static reflex *muscle* **inhibition** rather than reflex excitation. Thus, *this* **negative** *stretch reflex* opposes the shortening of the muscle in the same way that the **positive** stretch reflex opposes lengthening of the muscle. Therefore, one can begin to see that **the stretch reflex tends to maintain the status quo for the length of a muscle**.

When it comes to muscle movement, the negative stretch reflex automatically turns one muscle off when its opposing muscle is activated. This regulation is the process that results in fluid mobility.

Here, Sherrington's Law is helpful. This law states that *when a muscle receives a nerve impulse to contract, its antagonist simultaneously receives an impulse to relax.*

Basically, this describes *how* the body moves. Take walking, for example. First the front hip flexor quad muscle activates to lift the leg up and the leg steps forward. But in order for the leg to successfully lift, the back hamstring has to deactivate and turn off. If it remained on, the leg could not lift because the back hamstring would pull it down. So, in order for the body to move, the nervous system continually turns one muscle on, while at the same time turning another muscle off. The better the nervous system does this, the better balance it maintains. Balance is once again the overriding factor.

Determining the Type of Response

A sudden shortening of muscle fibers will trigger either positive or negative stretch reflexes, depending on the stimulus and intensity.

When things are balanced, a negative stretch response is stimulated. This response happens when one muscle turns on and it signals another muscle to turn off. It's a series of checks and balances. For example, when a football receiver runs a pass pattern the activation of the front quad muscles to lift the leg will automatically cause the hamstring on the back of the leg to relax. The moment the leg hits the ground the back hamstring muscles will activate to support the upright posture and the quads will automatically turn off and relax. The motions are fluid and efficient.

When the nervous system is unbalanced, and compensation layering is affecting the muscles, a positive stretch response triggers an FFF survival mechanism to take control of the situation. Here a snowball effect locks up one muscle after another. So when the same receiver attempts to run the same pass pattern, the hamstring will remain continually tight and be unable to relax sufficiently when the front quad is activated to lift the leg. Suddenly that tight hamstring gets pulled and the athlete is out of the game and more than likely out of action.

Chapter 7: Structure and Pain: The Role of the Hips and the Kinematic Chain

Hip Instability and Body Pain

Hip instability is a main contributor to chronic body pain. For years I had a hard time believing this. Through the functional neurological methods I practice, I am continually challenging the structural integrity of the body in order to detect patterns of weakness so adjustments can be made. What convinced me were the changes brought about for thousands of patients who demonstrated core pelvic weakness behind their back pain, headaches, tight hamstrings, sore shoulders, and you name it.

> ...man walks in an upright position and his limbs have become straightened to the point that almost no muscular strength is required to maintain the weight of the body against gravity. For instance, the direct line between the center of mass of the body and the direction of gravitational pull runs slightly behind the axes of the hip joints so that gravity tends to extend the hips and so that the ligaments of the hip joints, rather than the muscles, support the body against gravity. (708) (Guyton, Textbook of Medical Physiology, Fifth Edition 1977)

Remember, ligaments are supposed to hold the bones together, while muscles are designed to move the bones, and move the body. When ligaments turn into stretched out rubber bands, the muscles are forced to be continually tight while pulling double duty by taking over the role of the ligaments. One burned out muscle can cause a snowball effect to recruit other muscles for movement and to hold the body together, which they are not designed to do.

In order to detect which muscles are compromised in this way, I employ a very practical form of functional neurological testing. First the patient is properly positioned. Then firm pressure is placed against an isolated muscle at a very distinct angle to determine the quality of its immediate and precise contraction. The muscle needs to be isolated so it can be determined if muscle strength is the result of a group or individual muscle.

If not fully functioning, the muscle will weaken under testing and this shows that the nervous system's ability to completely activate the muscle is compromised.

What's actually being tested here is the efficiency of the signal that comes from the brain through the nerves to encourage full muscle activation. If it's an accurate signal there will be a muscle lock where the patient is holding strong against resistance. This is what I call a successful muscle lockout. If the muscle has been fatigued and cannot resist direct pressure, you can rightfully conclude that the muscle is carrying the burden of continual firing with minimal rest. When exacting pressure is brought to bear at a precise angle on such a muscle, it becomes shaky or even dynamically weak.

Once a successful lockout is established, the test is over for that specific muscle. This form of functional neurological testing should not be confused with traditional physical therapy muscle testing which only determines muscle strength, not isolated muscle weakness at the point of activation.

What I have found extremely interesting is that when pelvic weakness is present, sustained pressure on different parts of the body as well as quick shocks to the system will often compromise and weaken the integrity of the entire body. I understand that the reader is not getting the full experience of this, and reading about it is equal to reading about how to ride a bike. Unless you do it, you will never understand. For many, in order to understand this fully they would have to experience it for themselves. It is not only dramatic but it is inarguable. A demonstration of this technique can be found on my website **drmikeiz.com**.

During an assessment, while the patient is in a neutral position, their muscles can withstand numerous pressures from multiple directions. But the nervous system will show a positive reading to continual tension if I directly challenge and put strategic pressure on muscle or fascia attached to a weakened pelvis.

When treating patients, will every patient complaining about specific or generalized muscle pain have ligamental laxity at the pelvis? No, of course not. However, when a doctor or practitioner familiar with this possibility tests and finds a positive indicator for pelvic ligamental laxity, you better believe that their chronic aches and pains are the direct result of this hidden body instability. The practitioner who understands how the body hides both its weaknesses and injuries will always look for pelvic instability.

When treatment adds pelvic stabilization, the pain may come back within that generalized area, but it will present in another way. Athletes and patients often report strange muscle tightening in a different area of the body when they are seen during a course of treatment to correct their structural integrity. At first, this can be confusing to the patient. However, when you understand how everything within the body is connected it makes perfect sense. What transpires is that, once the pelvis regains its stability, the nervous system is able to relax and utilize body muscles more in line with normal patterns. When this happens, muscles which had been enslaved for long periods of time (sometimes years) to help shoulder the burden for weakened synergistic (nearby) muscles are suddenly liberated, and are once again allowed to contract according to their optimal design. That's the good news.

The bad news is that for a long time these muscles became accustomed to contracting in an improper pattern doing an inappropriate job. Also, sectors of these muscles may be atrophied, due to not fully and correctly firing. Newly freed, there will be a slight soreness when these now contract in the correct way. To keep athletes or patients from worry, I tell them they will feel like they helped a friend move. That slight soreness in weird places typically only lasts for about a day. I tell them to celebrate that because suddenly their body is now working more in line with how it always should have worked.

Deeper Into Anatomy and Pain

We touched briefly on anatomy earlier in this book, but now I want to take you a little bit deeper into the interconnectivity of the body and how this relates to imbalance and pain conditions.

My experience with thousands of patients has shown me that the cause of most sports injuries and non-sports related chronic pain results from a core hip imbalance, due to the ligaments of the pelvis weakening past a point of functional elasticity.

Because of this, when the painful area is treated and discomfort is relieved using established medical protocols, it might not be totally eliminated at its true source. Sometimes the same pain and physical restriction returns to that area or another pain arises close by bringing with it a slightly different physical restriction. Unfortunately for an athlete, this could lead to them being labeled "injury prone". In everyday life, patients are labeled as "chronic pain" sufferers.

Playing contact sports brings with it all types of minor and sometimes major trauma. Almost every injury sustained comes with a diagnostic nametag and an associated experience. Take the lower back strain, when a baseball player swings the bat either too much or too forcefully, their back may tighten painfully. In football, current and ex-players relate times when a collision with another player leads to a neck stinger, which radiated pain all the way down the arm. The point is that in sports we think linearly, relating the condition to what *appears* to be the most immediate cause. Consequently, doctors and trainers unknowingly sharpen this limited perspective based upon the precise training they are taught in regards to the best way to rehab specific injuries.

If an athlete's nervous system and ligamental structure ran more optimally, then the baseball player would experience greater elastic potential and the back strain would merely be slight soreness when waking up the next morning. In the case of the football player, no matter what, a hard hit is a hard hit, and it hurts. However, the more elasticity present within that athlete's body, the less muscle tightening would result after the traumatic hit. Thus, their ability to adapt goes up, while their chance for sustained injury goes down.

Carried deeper, muscles connecting on one end of the pelvis, often attach to multiple points down the leg, especially on either side of the knee joint. In order for a person to walk, or to sprint and quickly turn, these knee joint muscles must fire precisely to stabilize the joint and move the knee and leg evenly. When the nervous system is stuck in defensive mode, often there will be an over-contraction on one side of the joint and an unequal under-contraction on the other side.

For example, if a jogger's knee was compromised in this way, they would complain of knee pain after a run. In the case of a football running back this uneven situation could be tragic. Imagine that, on getting the ball, he suddenly sees a defenseman about to tackle him. The instant the running back plants his foot and quickly turns by twisting at the knee to avoid the tackle, an over-contracted inner knee muscle could suddenly contract so hard that the inner ACL (anterior cruciate ligament) and/or the middle meniscus could suddenly pull or tear. This is an all too common situation in football, basketball and soccer.

The Ongoing Pelvic Instability Problem

Once instability becomes prevalent within the pelvis, that triggers an alarm mechanism within the nervous system, where all muscles that can assist in balancing any unsteady joints are automatically activated. This is because one tight muscle will create a cascade of other tight muscles in order to maintain **stability, as in the positive reflex response.** Within that chronic state of emergency, the nervous system is programmed to keep muscles tight, and the upkeep of all connective tissue is put on hold. As the viscoelastic property of the ligaments stretch past certain set elastic points, all ligaments throughout the body weaken because the body's effort is focused on keeping muscles continually tight in order to maintain balance.

For athletes, they progressively lose the ability to "bend without breaking", and find themselves nursing a continually mounting set of minor injuries, or unfortunately a major one.

In order to correct this issue, the first step the doctor or practitioner must take is to stabilize the hip area. The concept of tissue stabilization is more than just my own personal clinical observation, it's an anatomical and physiological law discovered in the 1800's by an orthopedic surgeon named Henry Gasset Davis. In his honor, the characteristic viscoelastic behavior of connective tissue is called Davis's Law.

In a passage from Davis's 1867 book, *Conservative Surgery*, Davis pens:

> "Ligaments, or any soft tissue, when put under even a moderate degree of tension, if that tension is unremitting, will elongate....; "

> "When ligaments, or rather soft tissues, remain uninterruptedly in a loose or lax state, they will gradually shorten.... until they come to maintain the same relation to the bony structures with which they are united that they did before their shortening. Nature never wastes her time and material in maintaining a muscle or ligament at its original length when the distance between their points of origin and insertion is for any considerable time, without interruption, shortened." (Davis 1867)

The above passage explains the reason behind the success I have achieved with patients where other very competent doctors and physical therapists have been unable to get results. The first part of the quote states, "ligaments or any connective tissue under tension elongate." Under the properties of viscoelasticity, once this supportive ligament holding the pelvis together surpasses its elastic potential, it stretches past a point of immediate functional recoil.

Ligaments hold all bones together. The same connective tissue that make up ligaments can be found in tendons which connect muscle to bone. Since both are made up of connective tissue, they are all viscoelastic.

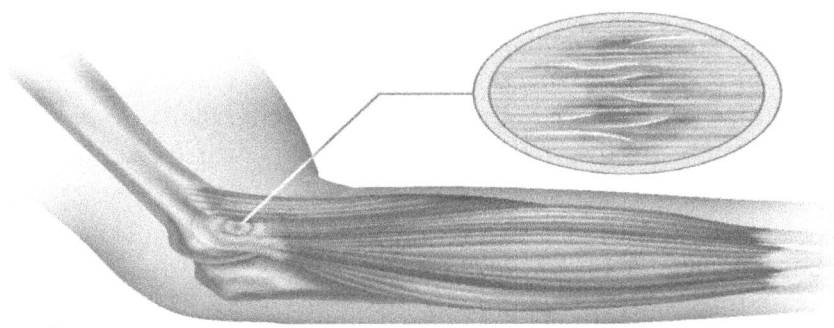

One Tendon Attaching Three Muscles to a Bone

Image 19

Let's explore what happens when a tendon becomes weakened. In the picture above, that slightly highlighted crisscrossing pattern indicates injury. Follow the line connecting the magnified image to the tendon highlighted by a slight bull's eye. That bull's eye highlights the very spot where the tendon has lost viscoelasticity. In other words, in that area the tendon became stretched out farther than it could functionally recoil (like a finger almost penetrating a garbage bag.)

Understand that each tendon possesses a certain "pull limit" whereby the attached muscle can contract and cause that muscle to move the bone. The moment this pull limit crosses the predetermined pounds per square inch limit, that triggers the nervous system to go on high alert. It knows that if that tension and pressure moves much farther past its preset safety limit, the tendon will rip off the bone. Put another way, tendons work on the concept of the "weakest link in the chain," where a chain, no matter how strong it appears, will break at its weakest link.

Now there is a transition from one situation to another, where the tendons require protection.

Muscles Protect the Tendons – An Unknown Truth

A primary purpose of the muscle is to protect the tendon. Muscles often defensively tighten when the nervous system perceives the possibility of a critical imbalance from tendon injury. To the nervous system this possibility is more than just an imbalance, it is a real emergency. As a result, its best and most direct response to prevent a tragedy is by overly tightening the muscle immediately connected to that tendon, as well as other close synergistic muscles to support that area. Once doctors, trainers, chiropractors and all other health care professions understand the foundational truth, the entire paradigm changes!

Across the board, most doctors and therapists treat tight muscles in a purely linear fashion. The muscle is treated directly according to the trauma it sustained and the pain the trauma produces. This means that whichever muscle is tight, the athlete or patient will receive a specific therapy primarily directed at relieving the tension within that muscle. As the tension relieves, the attention shifts to strengthening through rehab exercises.

Please understand I'm not saying there is something wrong or bad about various disciplines of massage, trigger point therapy, Active Release Technique, Graston soft tissue scraping, Rolfing, PNF stretching, and all forms of stretching, including yoga. These are all wonderful and effective techniques. And I am not saying you should no longer use these powerful techniques, I am only proposing that better results will be delivered first *if stability is brought to the body*, and then later the body is helped to regain its internal balance through the use of the body's own reflexes. Once this is done, many of the above techniques will then work even better than expected.

Another point to understand about why the body tightens the way it does is because of the way the nervous system pools all resources at once to achieve and maintain balance. Look at the above picture again and observe how three muscles share the same general origin attachment sites. The brachioradialis attaches to the distal lateral supracondylar ridge of the humerus. The extensor carpi radialis attaches to the lateral supracondylar of the distal humerus. Finally, the supinator attaches to the lateral epicondyle of the humerus.

The lateral epicondyle of the humerus (upper arm bone) is the part of the bone highlighted in the picture by the bull's eye. The word condyle means bump on the bone. Supra and epi are merely anatomy terms that mean above. Therefore, whether the description says supracondylar or epicondyle they essentially mean that all three muscles attach on the top part of that bone bump. Since all three muscles attach at the same point, the nervous system will pick up the tendon stretch and activate all three muscles at one time. This will lead to pain in different parts of the arm, elbow and forearm.

Getting to the Root of the Problem

Regardless of whether an athlete is competing at the high school, college, or professional level, the traditional treatment often used by trainers consists of lubricating the skin and scraping the fascia along the tightened region employing metal Graston scrapers which look like smoothed edged curved rulers. That technique, Rolfing, or even deep tissue massage addresses the overly tight fascia, while different popular techniques like Thai massage, trigger point therapy, ART (Active Release Technique), Muscle Re-education and PNF deal with the continual muscle tightness.

The problem with the above approaches is that they do not directly address the root issue. With tendons, the issue centers around the fact that when the body gets tight from continually holding some type of protective FFF contorted posture, there will be uneven pressure on certain specific areas of the body. In the skeleton, the weak link was ligaments holding the centralized pelvis together at the sacral iliac joint. When it comes to the muscular tendon attachment, the weak link can be anywhere in the body depending on how the body protectively defends itself.

Yes, Everything is Connected

The reason time was spent on the precise anatomical attachments of the above three muscles was to help you understand how tightly knit the body is. Since everything is connected, everything affects everything else.

When you go to a tennis club and see a bunch of people with Velcro straps around their forearms complaining of tennis elbow, their pain may not be the result of playing tennis. The extensor carpi radialis is used to extend the palm backwards (like a police officer telling a driver to stop). That motion causes the back of the hand to slightly extend at the end of the back-swing. However, the brachioradialis is primarily employed for arm flexion. Therefore, say a person attempts to lift a heavy box or they are handed an object too heavy for their bent arms to handle, the shock of that sudden over-contraction often strains the tendon attaching muscle to bone. Those muscles are aggravated when they play tennis and reach out with their racket to hit a backhand, but the pain likely resulted from the prior event.

Regardless of what shocked the muscle initially and caused it to over-contract, those three muscles share the same attachment site. Therefore much like the Three Musketeers' saying "All for one, and one for all," this event creates not only pain at the elbow, but *it weakens the action of all three of those muscles because all three will now be held within a continually contracted state in order to protect the now overly stretched tendon attachment to the bone.*

Adding insult to injury, in order for the newly tight muscles over the top of the forearm and the biceps region to either cramp or fail all together, the last major action the nervous system takes is to tighten the myofascial matrix (the fascia) covering that area. Now the area is not only sore but the fascia makes it tight. This tightness decreases range of motion. Since everything is connected, the increased tightness often creates more soreness, and/or the deep soreness creates greater tightness.

For example, in order for power lifters and football players to perform the clean and jerk maneuver, the athlete must first possess a powerful grip on the bar. Secondly, they must be able to transition the power wave from their legs through the upper body. In moving from the lower to the upper body, the biceps and brachioradialis must flex and the upper forearm muscles must contract in extension. Those are the primary transition maneuvers that, with core strength and stability, allow the bar to be lifted and successfully rest on the chest.

If one or all of the tendons are compromised, one or all of those muscles will not be as elastic, meaning they will not be as powerful. Worse still, since they all share the same attachment site, the nervous system will be forced to move past those three muscles and activate other muscles in an attempt to bring as much stability and power to that area as possible. This is because compensation creates both tightness and weakness in other areas of the body.

If you can look past the linear logic of one muscle, one pain; then you can successfully trace the pain back to its original cause, and fix it at the source. Regrettably, if the approach is linear, even though the athlete will leave the session with a degree of pain relief and a greater range of motion, the problem will return.

Transformation for Strains, Sprains and Pains via Compression

When muscular tendons become unsteady the condition is referred to as a *strain*. In the case of ligaments (connecting bone to bone), instability is referred to as a *sprain*. When a jogger unknowingly steps in a gopher hole, or trips over an object, and sprains their ankle or knee, typically they are prescribed a compression brace which securely fits over either their ankle or knee joint.

Why does compression over a joint work to allow the body to heal?

The answer can be found in Davis's Law. Abbreviated, this law states that ligaments, tendons, and fascia (all connective tissue), under strain, will elongate. Remember the concept of viscoelasticity and the stretched-out trash bag?

The only force that can ever pull against the tendon or the ligaments are the muscles. The breakdown of tendons and ligaments will result from either a constant chronic pull, a quick tug such as a football player being "blindsided," a sudden slip on ice or even being rear ended in a motor vehicle accident.

These quick forceful jolts create microtears within ligaments. Under these crises, the nervous system then overly activates surrounding muscles to secure the area through muscular verses ligamental strength. In time a cascade of multiple muscle and fascial tightening develops throughout the body, acting to pull on the body's central pelvic foundational core.

This will ultimately wind up pulling the hips apart like stretching the wall of a trash bag past its viscoelastic limits. Most of these situations result in the hips becoming destabilized, causing the nervous system to get locked into a continual state of FFF. Once a doctor, therapist or trainer addresses this, stabilization at the hip starts to reverse the situation allowing the nervous system to regain balance and optimal function.

The secret truth behind much of the unrelenting chronic pain people continually seek care for, actually originates from the multiple stressors of life constantly threatening the nervous system's ability to maintain optimal balance. Linear thinking keeps the average person going to their chiropractor for weekly or bi-weekly re-alignment adjustments. Others schedule massage sessions or additional therapies at appropriate intervals to stay on top of their pain. Exercise and yoga are further options to keep muscles artificially strong, but these are all efforts to address a problem that is in reality deeply structurally based. When pain fails to dissipate by these means, medical doctors prescribe pain medications and muscle relaxers along with physical therapy. If the pain continues, then stronger drugs and corticosteroids are employed. At this point the conversation turns towards nerve blocks and then surgery. Unfortunately, even with surgery, whether the inter-vertebral disk is shaved down, the vertebras are cut open or fused, or one entire hip is replaced, *neurologically based muscular imbalance is still active and present.*

Please understand that I am in no way advocating refusing surgery when it is necessary. When the body structure transitions to a point of degradation where it can no longer stabilize itself, you have to do what you have to do!

Whether it is a person that experiences pain at every attempt at standing, or an athlete who suddenly finds muscles continually tight, ninety percent of the time the cause is ligamental instability within the central pelvis, triggering a domino effect along kinematic chains, where different muscles become recruited to restore and maintain the best balance possible.

Chapter 8: The Process for Practitioners

Focusing on the Practitioner

This chapter is written for a specific audience, the practitioner. So, whether your specialty is in chiropractic, athletic training, physical therapy, structural integration, or any other modality typically employed to reduce pain, the steps laid out in this chapter will make your work more effective.

I find it ironic that a number of today's accepted therapies, designed to strengthen and improve range of motion, often wind up destabilizing the very defensive order the nervous system set up for the body's survival. When the body lacks firm stabilized support, today's established therapies are only capable of yielding short term gains for athletes. Many surface rehabilitative improvements which focus on enhanced coordination and relaxation of tight and defended muscles fade over time because progressive tightening is the result of unresolved neurological imbalances. By addressing only surface issues the practitioner leaves the nervous system still unbalanced.

Disturbingly, when compromised athletes reach exhaustion or push themselves because the game is on the line, they experience faulty play and unexpected injury. Instead of allowing an athlete to reach deep within to exert maximal effort during critical moments, an unbalanced nervous system perceives imminent danger. So instead of allowing the body to extend, open and speed up, the nervous system literally brakes, braces, and locks up. Continual play in this weakened condition often results in a decline in physical ability. Often, there's decline to a point where they are callously replaced by a younger player who may not necessarily be more talented, merely less neurologically burdened.

Of course, the extent of change that can be realized by the patient depends upon how defended and compromised the nervous system is before rehab therapies are performed. Too often as practitioners, we lose sight of Guyton's foundational statement:

"The most important ultimate role of the nervous system is to control the various bodily activities..."

"The major function of the nervous system is to process incoming information in such a way that *appropriate* motor responses occur." (pp 566-567) (Guyton, Textbook of Medical Physiology, Ninth Edition 1996)

Until practitioners consider assessment of the nervous system as the first and most important task, they will be unable to provide complete and lasting results for their athletes, patients or clients. Once you, in your field of expertise, place stability and nervous system balance as the first priority, you will find that much of the pain and restrictive patterns your athletes and patients struggle with are actually deeply ingrained survival habit patterns playing themselves out like classic vinyl records frustratingly repeating themselves due to a deep unseen scratch. When you deeply understand how to stabilize the physical structure and reset the nervous system, you will be amazed by how the body systematically and automatically returns itself back to higher states of optimized and pain-free function.

People must be re-introduced to the awesome power we each have within us to not only to heal, but to perform at a high level of ability. Too much pressure has been put on doctors to heal and trainers to train. Doctors, no matter their specialty, are successful *only to the extent they produce higher levels of stability within the patient's nervous system.* The greater the balance, the greater the healing. The same goes for athletic trainers and bodyworkers alike. The greater the neurological balance, the more stability which means advanced maneuvers can be performed with a decreased chance of injury. Because the movement potential becomes greater, there is more ability to bend without breaking.

This process is comprised of the following steps:
- Assessment
- Muscle Activation/Deactivation Completion
- Hip Stabilization
- Balance

Assessment

In order to assess the patient, the doctor or therapist must possess the ability to read the nervous system's functional neurological indicators of imbalance. They must also possess the practical knowledge of individualized reflexes which, when activated, serve as inner switches safely commanding specific areas of the body to reset. Every reset brings with it newer and greater levels of balance and body control.

To truly rehab an athlete or patient, the practitioner must first recognize the defensive pattern engaged, and secondly use the body's own reflexes to move muscles and muscle groups back to the neutral state. Remember the activation/relaxation cycle discussed earlier. Via influence from the nervous system some muscles can be stuck in a continual firing pattern, forcing the body to become tighter while others are stuck within a continual pattern of disengagement, becoming weaker. These patterns of engagement and disengagement occur in distinct layers. The more the layers present, the easier it is to challenge the nervous system in order to assess muscles.

Over many years of clinical practice, I have learned to recognize that there are typical patterns of protective muscular contractions that the nervous system locks the body into. In the assessment, I first see how compromised a person's nervous system is by determining how many muscular patterns of defense and compensation are currently activated and running. Remember the nervous system works by stimulus, *reflex,* response. Every challenge to body balance and stability forces the nervous system to reflexively activate and lock down a certain muscle or muscle/facial group to restore balance. Please refer to information previously presented on the kinematic chain which will explain this more in depth.

To see demonstrations of how an assessment is done, please see the videos on my website at **drmikeiz.com.**

In short, the assessment tests for patterns. The patient must be reassessed at the start of each office visit. As they regain neurological integrity, established patterns of self-defense begin to heal. As an example, say a patient is in full neurological defense with a portion of the body in full lock-down mode. I may have to activate five muscles impaired by the nervous system. As the patient improves, they will report that tightness and pain is decreasing. In follow-up treatments it becomes obvious the patient is improving because instead of five muscles displaying the defensive pattern in the assessment, I now find only three muscles affected.

Every layer stripped away blesses the patient with more ability to adapt to their environment through greater muscle control, less tightness, improved range of motion, and less pain within a short amount of time. The reason I say "a short time," is because deep healing comes from the nervous system regaining dynamic and full control of the body. There may be several layers of defense. In order to do this technique, the practitioner must be able to detect specifically which muscles are affected

Muscle Activation/Deactivation

Once the assessment determines what needs to be activated, it is extremely important to place the body in a position where the muscle group is in a state of contraction. For example, if the biceps muscle was causing the front of the arm to ache, then I would have the patient bend the arm at the elbow and further contract the biceps. This signals the nervous system to focus its attention on the biceps.

A tap or swipe of the body over that muscle is enough pressure to activate the mechanoreceptors. Recall earlier in the book the section about ion channels and the sodium/potassium pump. Its activation within the muscle will cause the brain to quickly fire the biceps muscle and complete the contraction. After that quick activation, the biceps muscle instantaneously moves through its resting stage and finally into a neutral position where it is primed, rested and ready to once again fully fire.

Here's what Guyton's says about stimulating over a compromised site:

> ...if a pain fiber is stimulated the person perceives pain no matter what type of stimulus excites the fiber. The stimulus can be electricity, heating the fiber itself, crushing the fiber, or stimulation of the pain nerve endings by damage to the tissue cells. Yet the person still perceives pain. (p. 584) (Guyton, Textbook of Medical Physiology, Ninth Edition 1996)

A second way to complete the contraction cycle is to forcefully stimulate over the muscle tendon attachment, then stretch it out fully for at least 20 seconds. Stretching confirms to the nervous system that there is no injury at that site, so it can then reset that muscle to its optimal length.

What we're actually doing is resetting tone. Muscles taken from the activation/deactivation state into relaxation become neutral and they can rest. The neutral state signals the brain to tell the muscle to move out of contraction. This resets a layer. Each layer requires resetting. Each reset brings with it a tone closer and closer to optimal.

Remember that for every muscle stuck in contraction there is a portion of another opposing muscle slightly incapacitated within a deteriorating state of atrophy. In the above example of biceps and triceps, the opposing muscle (triceps) must rest according to the activation/relaxation cycle. Once the nervous system has relinquished its hold on the biceps bringing it to its full contraction, that same energetic signal orders its opposite triceps muscle to complete its ongoing relaxation cycle and come back into a more favorable neutral position.

Note that the chronically contracted and relaxed muscles were brought back to neutral through the use of the body's own naturally occurring reflexes. Many accepted therapies today use tetanizing electrical current which contracts muscles so strongly they loosely exhaust, or dry needles which traumatize muscles, forcing the area into relaxation. Please bear in mind that I am not speaking out against these and other techniques which offer relief. I am only humbly suggesting that, according to the prime directive of the nervous system (survival at all costs), any procedures *past certain nervous system safety boundaries* will set up a recoil defensive action. Once that happens, the defensive nature of the nervous system will often make that new boundary tighter and stronger so that in the future when another "assault" happens, the body is more protected.

You will see that once you become familiar with how this process of peeling the proverbial neurological onion works, the athlete or patient will recognize other random symptoms that suddenly appear as confirmation that their nervous system is unwinding and becoming progressively unstuck. In this freer state, the nervous system feels safe to go deeper and deeper within the body in order to rebalance and heal areas shut down in the past. In truth, what comes up are old injuries that never fully healed. *As always, the nervous system took this course because survival takes precedence over precise function.*

Hip Stabilization

Most qualified doctors, chiropractors and other body therapy specialists get adequate to good results relieving surface pain and tension as well as promoting greater amounts of free motion and mobility through various techniques. However, if the treatment provided to the athlete or patient did not in some way focus on first bringing stability to the skeletal structure, then the treatment was incomplete because at some point the pain will come back in the exact same fashion.

Bodies are designed to be dynamically unstable. The more dynamically unstable a body is, the more adaptable it becomes. This means that whatever forces act against it, from a misstep to a physical collision, the healthy unstable body will absorb the impact and then quickly recoil back to a balanced centralized position. The dynamically unstable body bends without breaking.

When the body is structurally sound and dynamically pliable, all incoming forces create gradients directed towards the body's center, which, like a natural inner elastic spring, generates a vibrant recoil. This is how the nervous system maintains continual body balance. Healthy hip ligaments maintain the body's central stabilization and balance, yet allow it to move freely.

Now, with an improved understanding of what is really going on, I think you can better appreciate the genius of Dr. Davis in the 1800's.

The second part of his law states that when *"ligaments or any connective tissue maintains an uninterruptedly loose or laxed state, it will gradually shorten until it returns to its previously normal state"*. (Davis 1867)

The key to progressively resetting the nervous system back to optimal balance lies in stabilizing the skeletal structure with a sacroiliac belt. Proper assessment of the extent of hip ligamental laxity is crucial, and the practitioner must be trained in this area or they will be unable to accurately assess.

Bracing at the sacroiliac hip joint accomplishes two objectives. First, the way to tighten and restore ligaments back to optimal function is by instilling a state of slackness to the ligament. This stabilizes the condition outlined in Davis's Law. Once secured by a brace, previously stretched-out ligaments suddenly slacken and continually pulled tendons automatically start the process of shortening back to their original lengths as well as their original viscoelastic stretch potential. Since ligaments and tendons are thick and dense, this process takes time. Secondly, the moment the nervous system regains stability it automatically shifts out of FFF and acts upon changes that must be made to achieve long term healthy and rejuvenating results.

To stabilize the hips, I recommend my patients wear a Serola Biomechanic's sacroiliac belt for about three months. So far none have been pleased when hearing about this time length, but I then explain that most will be out of pain within about two weeks. However, I caution them that just because they no longer feel pain or discomfort, I highly recommend that they continue to wear the belt for the allotted three months allowing the body to transition from tightening the ligaments of the hip to tightening and securing the other ligaments holding their skeleton together.

Here is how the process works. Based on the multi-level compensatory nature of the nervous system, typically at two weeks their pain level will be down below the level of their conscious awareness. By this time the ligaments of the hip have tightened enough to satisfy a minimal stability requirement. This means that although the body is not completely stable, it is stable enough to no longer trigger pain. In reality, this improvement is only at about 80%.

The three-month time period of wearing the belt is a conservative period I have found to be most effective to help most patients fully recover. Honestly, I find that people are encouraged with the knowledge that as long as they provide their skeleton with this structural support they will move towards healing, and then they are typically understanding and willing to comply. Many get excited by the prospect that once they achieve the initial yet crucial partial stability of the hip, their body will actually start the process of balancing and healing other parts and areas they don't even know about, currently lying dormant. What happens is by the two to two and one-half month mark the nervous system has rebalanced as much of the body as it can and then at that point it will return to the original hip ligaments and tighten those to the full 100%.

Athletes will typically wear the belt when they are wearing regular clothes. When training or competing, they can wear compression shorts under their practice or game gear. At least that way their hips can maintain some semblance of core stability and support while their bodies are fully active.

The more stability and support the nervous system secures from the skeletal structure, the better it works. The better it works, the more it will acknowledge and address areas out of balance that are not in top working order. By maintaining the highest stability possible through the corrective phase, the nervous system will properly rebalance itself, providing the best opportunity to heal. Always remember, the body is self-regulating, and it is self-healing.

Balance: The Last Piece of the Puzzle

With the patients and athletes I treat, once they are structurally stabilized, and their nervous systems are reflexively reset as much or as deeply as their nervous system will allow for that session, the topic of balance training is discussed and taught. In order to assess ability, I ask patients to stand on one leg to determine how long they can successfully hold that position. At some point, of course, they will begin to wobble to regain stability. What's happening is that small muscles along the spine are not strong enough to maintain postural stability and dynamic function.

Smooth body motion starts with the activation of these small muscles which initiate motion then transitions to larger muscles which continue motion. When those small muscles are not working effectively, body dynamics and balance suffers.

To maximize balance, I advise patients to progressively challenge themselves by first standing longer periods of time on one foot, with eyes open, then later closed. Later they move on to more challenging exercises like balancing on varying types of wobble boards first with both feet, then later on one foot. Once wobble surfaces are mastered, left brain to right brain, and right brain to left brain exercises are performed by tossing objects from one hand to another while on the balance board. The last, most difficult, and the most superior form of balance training concludes when the patient is able to balance themselves on a slack line. A slack line is a flattened, webbed rope tied off at two surfaces. Think of it as a modern tightrope. When a person can balance themselves on such a small and yet highly movable surface, their nervous system has now reached a superior level of competence, and most importantly, exceptional adaptability.

Conscious control over balance is illusionary, because your ability to successfully balance on one leg is a direct reflection of how well your nervous system adapts to the environment. If you have trouble balancing on one leg, then rest assured your nervous system is over-worked and stressed. To simply stand still in place, your nervous system must very precisely activate and control muscle tension on either side of your body. Too much one way or the other tips your balance forward, backward or to the side. Every time you walk, you're balancing on one leg or the other. So don't take this information lightly.

There are two types of muscles. First are the prime movers. These are large muscles used for lifting weight, locomotion, and gross movement of the limbs. Stabilizers and rotators make up the second muscle type, and these are the ones most responsible for balance. As stabilizers, these very small muscles help ligaments and tendons to stabilize the body. As rotators they both initiate and control the refined movements necessary for precise and ordered movements.

The better the nervous system maintains balance, the more control it has over each of these individual muscles. For instance, when properly balanced and calm, all muscles, especially the small ones along the spine, turn fully on and then reflexively, fully off. These small muscles along the spine are exceptionally important for both balance as well as precise movements. Besides small stabilizers, their crucial role as rotators is often overlooked.

Muscles Along the Spine

Tight erector spinae group muscles are the cause of discomfort in a number of areas. Patients will complain of low back pain, restriction and soreness in the upper back, chronic neck and shoulder pain, and headaches. They may be afflicted in one or several of these areas. Some will blame time spent in front of the computer for their chronic neck and shoulder pain. Others will note the horrible headaches they feel at the base of the back of their skull. But all these different painful manifestations come from

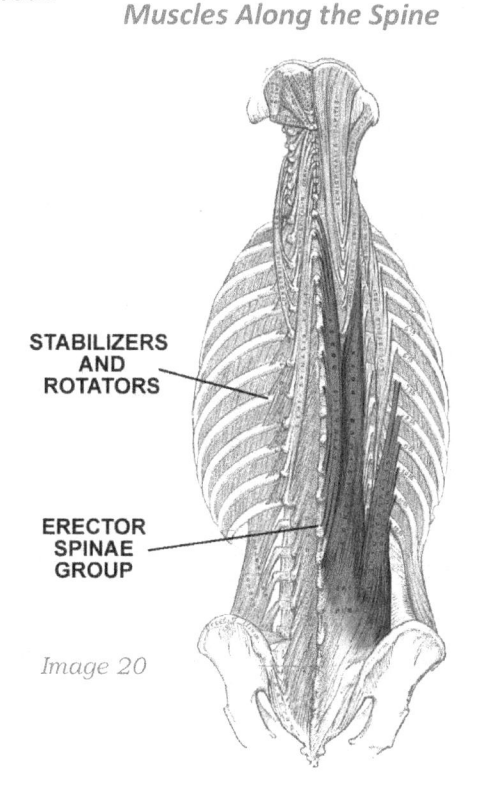

STABILIZERS AND ROTATORS

ERECTOR SPINAE GROUP

Image 20

the same source: a destabilized structure which has created an unbalanced nervous system.

In the image to the left, note the stabilizer and rotator muscles indicated. These smaller muscles are combined and layered to make up part of a structure which runs from the occiput to the sacrum called the erector spinae. The erector spinae group acts as a rope which allows for minor movements such as bending backwards and forwards and side to side. This group is not tasked with any finite movements, only gross motions.

For athletes these smaller muscles are more crucial than the bigger power muscles trained thorough strength and conditioning. Brute strength is trained. This strength comes from hard training of the prime movers, which make up our big muscles, like those in the chest, legs and arms. Speed, dexterity and finesse are developed. The finesse muscles are those small muscles previously discussed. While balance training makes them stronger, you must always remember, the nervous system has final authority on whether they partially or fully activate.

When you see athletes make spectacular and precise plays where their bodies gyrate and twist, you are

Body Rotation for Moving Forward

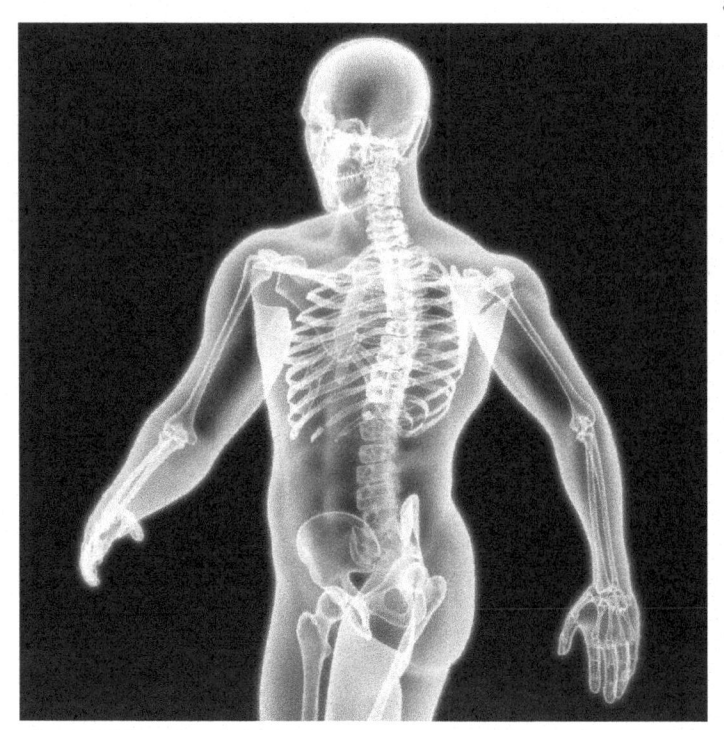

Image 21

seeing the effect these smaller muscles have on movement.

When these tiny muscles between each vertebra contract individually, the spine is free to perform what is called "coupled motion," or two motions in one. For instance, say the brain contracts the small muscles on the right side of the spine. These contractions cause the spine to lean and rotate right. Simultaneously, the muscles on the left side of the spine must de-activate allowing for this right lean and rotation to fully manifest.

Precise walking/running depends on the spine's ability to perform coupled motion. Specifically, this means that when the body steps to one side, the spine is able to rotate the torso to that side. Observe the body rotation picture and note how as the right foot steps forward, the body leans slightly to the right. For that split second, the body is off balance, falling laterally to the right. In order to counter that side lean, the torso rotates towards that right side.

At first, it seems like the body is working against itself. If it is already leaning right, why would it exaggerate the imbalance by then rotating further to the right? The answer is ingenious. Remember the kinematic chain running from the right groin to beneath the left shoulder? By rotating right, not only does the left arm swing forward in counterbalance to the right side, the nervous system successfully contracts the abdominal obliques ending under the left armpit, and upper left pectoral muscles which precisely counterbalance the right body lean. Simply put, the shoulder must precisely balance the opposite hip. You can tell the upper spine contracts by noting how the upper vertebral bones of the torso now slightly bend left. That upper leftward muscle contraction along with left torso rotation, is in fact a "perfect" counter-balance to the necessary right lean that is a natural consequence of stepping forward with the right foot. From that twisted position the body converts into a natural spring.

Neurological imbalance can be detected through gait assessment. In a patient lacking this spring, the tendency is to walk with a wider stance to make up for the imbalance. This forces the body to tighten muscles along the spine and in the torso to protect the brain from upward vibration caused by a thudding side to side gait. The greater the imbalance, the wider the stance. The wider the stance the more pronounced the "thud."

Part of the reason some structural bodyworkers are not aware of this is due to time constraints during medical training. Often anatomy classes make little mention of all the small muscles that, like rope fibers, make up the entire erector spinae group bundle. Since their small contractions seem insignificant, their crucial contribution to balance often goes unnoticed. Their individual actions are key drivers for the specific left, right, oblique and rotatory actions necessary for the nervous system to maintain the highest automatic level of balance possible. To the extent the brain activates FFF defensive measures, the nervous system loses precise control of these small muscles. The issue regarding all of the small muscles is that they not only stabilize the spine, they also act as stabilizers for every joint in the body. If you're hiking through the woods and an unstable rock slides under your foot, the mechanoreceptors within the ankle joint signal the nervous system to rebalance the body quickly in order to prevent a fall or sprain. The first muscles to activate are those small stabilizers right next to the joint. Ideally, their contractions will activate the bigger muscles of the lower leg.

The over-riding point is and always will be: the longer a person remains in FFF, the less all smaller muscles along the spine and next to the joints remain deactivated or not working at full potential. *Proper rehabilitation must always follow the order of first reactivating those smaller muscles and then strengthening the essential muscles controlling and coordinating autonomic/automatic balance.* As it stands today, most rehab exercises focus on strengthening the big prime movers, *often omitting the smaller stabilizers and rotators.*

Think back to the reflex response, when the hand moved away from the flame and caused a neurological pathway of pain (the second messenger) to develop in the tissues. Stiffness often results from too many reflex responses which lock muscles into continuous painful contractions.

Research has indicated the probability that reflexes of the small muscles along the spine can account for up to 42% of torso stability. (Kevin M

Moorhouse 2007) From what I have witnessed to date in patient response to balancing exercises that stimulate reflexive responses in these tiny muscles, this rings true. These exercises neurologically signal the tiny muscles to complete their locked and often painful contractions and move into relaxed states. The result is greater stability along with sounder structural alignment.

Once the nervous system is able to exercise better control over movement, the body benefits by moving one step closer to optimal function and greater adaptability. The more adaptable the nervous system becomes, the more adaptable the person is to the environment, which means they can function better during times of duress.

The goal for chronic pain patients and injured athletes is getting the nervous system to feel safe enough to allow proper rehabilitation and acceptable activation of muscles in order to bring a higher level of control and balance to the body. As long as the body lacks stability, any gains within these small and crucial muscles are short-lived. In the case of the erector spinae muscles lining the spine, as long as the nervous system is forced to be continually vigilant, those smaller muscles will cease their individual functions and instead act as a continual tight rope from the triangular sacral base at the bottom of the hip all the way to the occiput bone at the base of the skull. The tighter it gets the more impossible it is to walk with a natural rotation. The patient will walk with a more pronounced side to side walk. Not only will their ability to balance be compromised, but the more out of balance they get, the tighter that huge spinal rope becomes.

Pain During the Healing Process

As discussed previously, sometimes a patient will experience pain in a different area as they go through this course of healing. As tight muscles are neurologically reactivated, the body changes. It now has a "new normal", which is in actuality a "more correct normal". Previously tight muscles can feel tired and sore, while previously disengaged muscles will typically feel discomfort similar to the feeling of working out a muscle in the gym that has not been worked out in a while. As the body regains its attribute of dynamic instability, it is engaging the proper muscles required for balance.

When this happens, a patient may express a sense of worry and concern that they are now stricken with a new predicament. I comfort them by informing them that that change is a validation their body is truly healing because it is now strong enough to make changes it dared not make in the past when stuck in patterned layers of survival. I tell them *it is not something new that just came on, it is something old that just came up.*

Usually many of the spontaneous body discomforts come up at the beginning of treatment. Later on, the patient notes pleasant changes as their nervous system assumes greater control over the body, making the body more adaptable. As they progress, I often tell the patient in fun that the better they get, the harder they are making me work to find the weakness.

The length of time this unraveling process takes depends on how long the patient has been compromised. Compared to a typical course of traditional chiropractic therapy, treatment length is not long at all, and usually lasts two to three months. In addition, the patient will not have to come in for as many frequent visits. Each visit is a therapy session with a pre-determined goal of restoring function to the next presenting layer of nervous system dysfunction.

This is what makes my practice enjoyable. Every patient on every visit is a like a new patient because the body is always changing to continually adapt to the environment in a different way as it heals. The more restrictions removed from the patient, the healthier they become. Within the world of athletics, the more imbalances are corrected, the stronger, faster, and more dexterous the athlete becomes. More importantly as athletes are more powerful today than ever before, the better the athlete is able to take a hit and bounce back, the better they will be able to concentrate and perform movements they trained hard to accomplish and perfect.

Always remember this, the body must first feel a certain level of structural stability before it will allow itself to return to its optimal settings where muscles activate and de-activate on time and in perfect synchronicity. The closer the nervous system returns to this peak level of control, the more it returns to its maximal self-healing potential. Think of healing not as a sprint, but rather a marathon. Every defensive compensation stripped away should be celebrated. The more that gets stripped away, the greater the reduction in pain and physical restriction.

Sports Rehabilitation and Chronic Pain Management

Because of the many successes thousands of my patients have been able to achieve, I believe this book offers a better way of rehabilitation and pain management. I've seen countless individuals that have tried a myriad of modalities to alleviate symptoms. This approach instead promotes true healing in the body. As a **structural bodyworker or sports trainer**, you can work smarter instead of harder by concentrating your efforts on the nervous system. By stabilizing the body and restoring neurological balance, you will find that the nervous system will work with you and no longer against you. You will find your results will improve, because instead of holding on for dear life, the newly restored nervous system will find new challenges invigorating instead of threatening. Remember, we are made to adapt. Every adaptation is looked upon by the nervous system as a new way to survive. The key is, and always will be, to make it safe for the nervous system to open up and accept the changes you introduce.

The beauty of this approach is one where you can use your existing training in order to facilitate improvement. You don't have to learn any new techniques. Just by putting the nervous system first or at least making its balance a high priority through whatever training or rehabilitation programs you currently engage in, will bring you success. Once the nervous system is stabilized and progressively rebalanced, your wonderful and established training regimens will work exceptionally better.

Now it is time to see for yourself.

Conclusion

For too long people have associated tight bodies and muscles as expected and inescapable realities of old age. In athletics, tight bodies and tight muscles are categorized negatively as consequences of playing hard, and positively as natural results of intense strength training. The way forward, either for an athlete or someone seeking to live in as mobile and pain-free a body as possible, is to bring greater awareness to the way we currently heal our bodies. The assumption that the problem is gone when the pain is gone is the biggest fallacy in sports medicine.

Now that you know the real difference between a tight body and a strong one, it is my sincere intention that you take the message of this book to heart. The vast majority of people who seek pain relief find that medicine can only offer symptom relief, and not true healing. They assume the problem is taken care of only to find it resurfacing later. Over time, often more extensive measures must be taken to gain relief. Some get to the point where they're told nothing more can be done and they must learn to live with pain as a constant companion. In the meantime, quality of life has suffered as they are forced to gradually eliminate doing the things that bring enjoyment and value to living.

I implore you to seek quality healing, by understanding that symptoms which motivated you to seek professional help are in reality just the tip of the iceberg and that you can become whole again. True healing as well as maximal optimization of the nervous system is possible. The body strives to gain balance. It just needs a little help to heal sometimes.

The process of true healing requires some time. Most people accept that, given their final results. When one layer of compensation is stripped away, the nervous system needs a little time to reorient and then reactivate itself now that it's working from a higher-level perspective. The more the layers are stripped away, the more overall muscle control is returned to not only the big prime movers but more importantly the smaller stabilizers and rotators.

Once balance and muscle activation are re-established and the nervous system progressively works at greater rates of competency, adjustments must be made where imbalances appear. For that you need a practitioner familiar with the methods of testing and correcting the nervous system through functional neurology.

I cannot say how many layers deep any person's compensations go, because I don't know the complete history of any person's life other than my own. So there's no way to know how many total treatment sessions are needed for any individual. But patients find as they go through this process, that as we give the body support to heal itself, significant improvements happen. Pain lessens or is eliminated, mobility and dexterity increase, moods heighten and lighten, and overall life becomes better.

This is true healing.

Patient Testimonials

Martin: Severe Back Pain After Playing Basketball

I am a 38-year-old, healthy man. I play basketball three times a week, go for walks with the family, and do push-ups and sit-ups for strength training. I am 5'11" and weigh about 180 pounds. I am not overweight. However, despite all of this, twice over the past couple of years, I threw out my back out while playing basketball.

When I say "threw out" my back, I truly mean that, because I don't know what even happened. One moment, I'm running, jumping, passing, shooting, etc., and then all of a sudden, I have a severe, sharp pain in my lower back which leads to pain in other parts of the back. Due to the blood flow and adrenaline, I was able to finish playing basketball; but after getting in the car and driving home, I could barely get out of my car due to the pain. Walking and any type of movement was very, VERY painful.

The first time this happened, I went to work that morning, but again, I could barely get out of my car...or walk, or sit, or stand for that matter. I immediately called my chiropractor, Dr. Mike, and luckily, he had an opening that afternoon. Dr. Mike assessed me and adjusted me and said that it actually wasn't my back that was the problem, but my hips that were out of line. He gave me a stabilizing belt to wear under my clothes and honestly, the next day I was probably almost back to perfect health and I had no more back pain. I was back to playing basketball the next week.

The second time this happened, the pain wasn't quite as severe on day one, but nonetheless, I could not walk without pain, I couldn't play basketball and I had to sit and stand up very gingerly. Of course, I called Dr. Mike and while the results were not "instantaneous" like they were the first time, eventually with adjustments, wearing the hip stabilizing belt again, and taking the proper supplements, within a few weeks, I was able to get back to what I had always normally done (playing basketball, going for walks, push-ups, etc.). Today I do not live in any chronic pain, back or any other. My wife and I are very thankful to have Dr. Mike in our area and to have his expert professional counsel in areas such as this. -*Martin Hale*

From Sports Injury to Athletic and Personal Success

Dr. Mike single handedly saved my athletic career. I was an athlete that did not take care of my body in the way that I should have, and pursuing my aspirations of being a professional athlete would not have been possible if it were not for Dr. Mike. Dr. Mike has saved me months, if not years, from being on the sidelines.

I am a soccer goalkeeper and I have a second tryout with a MLS team in Atlanta in December. With training at a higher level, I have had a variety of injuries ranging from nagging minor injuries to very serious injuries. Every time I have picked up an injury I have gone to Dr. Mike, and every time he has cut the time I would be sidelined injured at least in half.

Dr. Mike got my body in the proper alignment, and not only made me a better athlete, but a better person. Getting me on the proper supplements and nutrition has made me a healthier person, mentally and physically. I owe a lot of my success to Dr. Mike, not just in sports but in business as well.

Dr. Mike taught me how to use a balance board to my advantage by showing me exercises and drills on how to trigger and train my left brain and right brain to work together as one. Since Dr. Mike showed me this important drill, I cannot recall giving up a terrible rebound that lead to a goal, instead I have swallowing up every belted shot with the greatest of ease. There are plenty of facets to goalkeeping that come more naturally to me because Dr. Mike showed me this vital drill.

Dr. Mike didn't just put me on the road to recovery, he put my life back on track. Anytime an athlete suffers a serious injury its unbelievably difficult on them mentally. I was beyond depressed with my injury, I honestly thought it was over. Dr. Mike believed in me and told me that if I believed in him, believed in his philosophy and most importantly believed in myself that I would come back even stronger. I put my faith in him and his vast knowledge and my faith was rewarded. He helped me physically, mentally and spiritually.

-Peter M. Krafcik

Fayne: Great Results from Compression Belt

I have been seeing Dr. Mike Izquierdo for 8 years. He is a brilliant chiropractor and a nutritionist who always has something new to share with you. He's always learning, researching and discovering more about the practice of healing.

One thing that I will always thank Dr. Mike for is the Serola Biomechanic's belt. The little bit of compression from this belt around my hips, provides enough structure that it allows my body to stop compensating with other muscles. It is very calming and allows my body to relax and get back to normal. Sciatica? Belt. Tipped pelvis? Belt. It's great. I am into a lot of activities that sometimes knocks me off my feet, sailing, curling, hiking... The belt helps a lot.

-Fayne Copeland

Thirty Years of Pain GONE After One Visit!

Words cannot communicate how thankful I am to this belt. People would always ask me why I never sat down. The reason was because it hurt! I had to keep standing and walking to keep the pain at bay. I had never been the same since being hit head on 30 years ago, and spending 2 ½ weeks in a coma. Occupational therapy gave me all types of rehab exercises, but in the long run, nothing worked so I learned to live with the pain.

At first, I was skeptical when Dr. Mike told me the cause of the low pain I had been suffering with for 30 years was actually from my hips. Although his explanation made sense, 30 years of pain makes a person really pessimistic. I hoped it would help, but I didn't have much faith.

On the second visit, even Dr. Mike could not believe my results. The pain was gone, and I was able to comfortably sit down again. Dr. Mike warned me that parts of my now newly stabilized body had to be balanced and strengthened. I told him I was OK with that. Personally, I didn't care. I am just amazed at how that belt and whatever Dr. Mike did caused that excruciating constant pain to be finally gone.

-*Dawn Feckner*

Alice Can Now Sleep Through the Night!

I used to have incredible pain so bad that I could barely sleep at night. I even went to New York to see a doctor who specialized in a therapy similar to dry needling. After several treatments with this doctor, which did not help the pain, I finally gave in and got a low back facet laminectomy. After the surgery the pain continued. I found this devastating and thought that I might have to learn to live with this.

Then I met Dr. Mike. After using the belt and having the muscles balanced, I felt enough relief that I could sleep through the night. Prior to seeing him I had experienced this pain for over four years. I'm also walking much better with less pain during the day, and can walk for longer periods without resting. In fact, my daughter and I have spent up to two full hours out walking.

Now that I'm coming in only for maintenance care, I continue to wear the belt rarely, and only during times when I feel unsteady. At 90 years of age, I'm much steadier than friends my age and I know it's all due to the balancing work. I'm grateful for the results I have achieved from your care.

- *Alice McGinty*

Fifteen Years of Back Pain Eliminated for Fellow Chiropractor

Dr. Mike has been a friend of mine for over fifteen years. During that time, I have continued with pain in my sacroiliac and across the lower lumbar spine which I have treated with various forms of chiropractic. I myself have been a chiropractor for 25 years and could not find relief that would last.

In January I spoke to him about the condition and the imbalances which I found in my core. Thanks to his good treatment and care and the use of the Serola belt I was able to achieve the ability to regain my flexibility and live without the pain I had previously had. It all had to do with getting a balance between being mobile and staying stable.

I had to stop weight lifting and running years ago because of the pain. Thanks to the change in my condition I am now bike riding three times a week and doing light workouts with my son. After manipulation and the Serola belt have now been applied, I have achieved flexibility and strength in only 90 days that I haven't seen in years. My only regret is that I didn't do this before.

-*Scott Van Oosten D.C.*

Fitness Buff Sees Marked Improvements

After seeing Dr. Mike regularly for a few months now, I feel better, physically and mentally, than I have in over 10 years. He helped reset my nervous system to run the way it's intended to run. Seeing and feeling those changes has helped me keep my end of the bargain as nothing comes for free. My running has improved, along with the workouts, weight loss and core strength. I'm very grateful and will definitely be back for regular visits.

-*Kelly Timmerman*

"You Don't Have Back Problems"

I had been diagnosed with bulging discs and was facing back surgery. Dr. Mike noticed I was walking and standing crooked, ran some diagnostics, made an adjustment, and prescribed a Serola Sacroiliac Belt for me to wear. I'll never forget his words, "you don't have back problems; it's your hip". It's been 3 years and I did not require back surgery. Thank God, Dr. Mike, and the belt.

-René R. Fonseca, PMP, MBA

After Spinal Fracture, a Balanced and Healed Body

For almost ten years now, I have known Dr. Mike Izquierdo. During the course of these years I have faced the obstacles of a sacral spinal fracture, an over the counter medicine causing dangerous side effects to my organs, lymphatic and adrenal fatigue, and the effects of stress.

I can honestly say that I don't know where my body or I would be without Dr. Mike. I have watched my body through his guidance come to balance, heal itself, and find an overall better quality of life. Dr. Mike is a genuine, caring, and tremendously talented holistic doctor. I continue to learn from him and use this knowledge and experience in my own practice.

I highly recommend taking the time to see him…it will change your life.

- Theresa Eckman LMT, CIRM, ECYT, CMRT, KHFRM, Founder of Wholistic Healing in Northfield, Ohio

Glossary

Activation/Relaxation Cycle: Based on Sherrington's Law, when one muscle turns on (facilitates or activates), the opposing muscle turns off (inhibits or relaxes).

Balance: The ability of a body to maintain stability in a gravitational field.

Chronic Pain: Pain that persists past normal healing time. Pain is usually regarded as chronic when it lasts or recurs for more than three months.

Connective Tissues: Ligaments, fascia, and tendons.

Defended Muscle: A muscle stuck in a continuous state of contraction.

Elasticity: The natural recoil ability of both muscle and connective tissue. When optimally functioning, it gives both patients and athletes the ability to bend but not break.

Fight/Flight/Freeze (FFF): The range of common nervous system survival reactions to stress.

Flow: A unique psychological state during which a subject becomes completely absorbed in a task. For example, when an athlete is in flow, they report that they associate this focused state of attention with several factors which can include heightened senses, a sense of oneness, feelings of total control, and feelings of being "in the zone".

Hebb's Rule: Synaptic conductivity changes as a result of repetitive firing. Hebb's rule can be summarized as "nerves that fire together, wire together.

Hilton's Law: This law states that a nerve that enervates a muscle will also enervate the skin overlaying it in addition to a joint located beneath it.

Layers of Compensation: Tiered, multiple layers of buried stress, built up over the course of months and years. The younger the person, the more punishment and compensations their body can handle without conscious awareness of anything wrong.

Ligamental Laxity: When ligaments are stretched past their ability to recoil and hold structural integrity.

Ligaments: Connective tissue responsible for holding the skeletal structure together. Ligaments join bones to bones. They characteristically have the property of viscoelasticity, which means once stretched past a certain point the tissue loses the ability to recoil back.

Muscle Atrophy: The wasting away of a muscle due to disuse. Disused muscles become weaker and eventually begin to shrink.

Muscle Firing: The neurological activation or triggering of muscle movement.

Muscle Tone: The continuous state of muscle activation, ideally at around the sympathetic resting rate of 1 Hz, which allows the body to stay upright, calm, and ready to move and properly adapt to the outside environment at a moment's notice.

Neurology: The science which explains the methods used by the brain, spinal cord and nerves to communicate messages that promote the adaptation of the body to the environment.

Nervous System: The brain, spinal cord and nerves that exit from the cord which relay environmental information to the brain. The communication system which allows the body to adapt to the outside environment. The ultimate role of the nervous system is to control various body activities achieved by controlling skeletal muscle contraction.

Proprioceptive Neuromuscular Facilitation (PNF): Stretching technique utilized to improve muscle elasticity which has been shown to have a positive effect on active and passive range of motions. This stretching should ideally be done after competition or exercise, but never before.

Stabilization Muscles: Small "finesse" muscles, mainly those located next to the spine and joints, that allow for fine movements of the physical body.

Stress: A force acting against the balancing mechanism of the nervous system. It takes three forms. Physical stress comes from trauma (i.e. a fall or hit). Mental-emotional stress typically comes from having to meet deadlines and commitments or negative human interaction. Chemical/toxic stress results from exposure to toxic chemicals or the consumption of overly processed, non-nutritious foods which forces the body to detoxify while simultaneously trying to extraction any nutrition possible.

Tendons: Connective tissue which attach muscle to bone.

Turned-off Muscle: An underactive or under recruited muscle which cannot be contracted because the message is not effectively getting from the brain to the muscle.

Viscoelasticity: A property of any substance that is concurrently viscous and elastic. When pressure is put on a viscoelastic material, it has the ability to rebound to its original shape. However, with sustained pressure past a certain point, it deforms.

References

Cantu, Robert I., and Alan J. Grodin. 1992. *Myofascial Maniplation Theory and Clinical Applicaton.* Gaithersburg: Aspen Publishers, Inc.

Chang, Seoyon Yang and Min Cheol. 2019. *Chronic Pain: Structural and Functional Changes in Brain Structures and Associated Negative Affective States.* June 26. Accessed 8 14, 2020. https://www.ncbi.nlm.nih.gov/pmc/articles/PMC6650904/.

Csikszentmihalyi, Mihaly. 1990. *Flow: The Psychology of Optimal Experience.* New York: Harper Colins Publishers.

Dahlhamer J, Lucas J, Zelaya, C, et al. 2016. *Prevalence of Chronic Pain and High-Impact Chronic Pain Among Adults — United States.* Accessed 8 11, 2020. http://dx.doi.org/10.15585/mmwr.mm6736a2 .

Davis, Henry G. 1867. *Conservative Surgery as Exhibited in Remedeying Some of the Mechanical Causes that Operate Injurously Both in Health and Disease.* New York: D. Appleton & Company.

Demange MK, Fregni F. 2011. *Limits to clinical trials in surgical areas.* Accessed 8 2020. https://www.ncbi.nlm.nih.gov/pmc/articles/PMC3044561/ .

Duhigg, Charles. 2014. *The Power of Habit: Why We Do What We Do in Life and.* New York: Random House.

Goldman, Charles. 2020. *Contract breakdown for Chiefs QB Patrick Mahomes' extension.* 7 7. Accessed 8 2020. https://chiefswire.usatoday.com/2020/07/07/kansas-city-chiefs-qb-patrick-mahomes-contract-breakdown-base-salary-bonus-salary-cap/.

Guyton, Arthur C. and Hall, John E. 1977. *Textbook of Medical Physiology, Fifth Edition.* Philadelphia: W. B. Saunders Company.

—. 1996. *Textbook of Medical Physiology, Ninth Edition.* Philadelphia: W. B. Saunders Company.

John D. Loeser, MD , et al, ed. 2000. *Bonica's Management of Pain.* Philadelphia: Lippincott Williams & Wilkin.

Kevin M Moorhouse, Kevin P Granata. 2007. "Role of reflex dynamics in spinal stability: intrinsic muscle stiffness alone is insufficient for stability." *Journal of Biomechanics* 1058-65.

Lubinger, Bill. 2019. "Remember when ... off-season was work time for the Cleveland Browns (and all pro athletes)?" *cleveland.com.* January 12. https://www.cleveland.com/browns/2010/05/remember_when_off season_was_wo.html.

Meyers, Thomas W. 2001. *Anatomy Trains: Myofascial Meridians for Manual and Movement Therapists.* First. Edinburgh: Churchill Livingstone.

National Institute on Drug Abuse. 2020. *Opioid Overdose Crisis.* 5 27. Accessed 8 2020.

National Institutes of Health. 2014. *Pain: Hope Through Research.* January. Accessed 8 2020. https://www.ninds.nih.gov/Disorders/Patient-Caregiver-Education/Hope-Through-Research/Pain-Hope-Through-Research.

NFL Football Operations. 2015. *Evolution of the NFL Player.* January 17. https://operations.nfl.com/the-players/evolution-of-the-nfl-player/.

Sharman, et al. 2006. "Proprioceptive neuromuscular facilitation stretching : mechanisms and clinical implications." *PubMed.* https://www.ncbi.nlm.nih.gov/pubmed/17052131.

Image Citations

Image 1: *PNF Stretching Technique* by Shutterstock

Image 2: *Ligaments Connect Bones to Bones* by Scie Pro - Shutterstock

Image 3: *Everything, in Some Way, Goes Through the Hips* by Serola Biomechanics, Serola.net

Image 4: *Exaggerated Defended Posture* by Oleksii, Ovchynnikov – © rf123.com

Image 5: *The Hand Moves Away from the Flame* by NoPainNoGain - Shutterstock

Image 6: *Abdominal Obliques Connecting to Ribs* by 3D4Medical from Elsevier

Image 7: *A Kinematic Muscle Chain* - Public Domain

Image 8: *Extracellular Matrix* by QuynhAnhDs - Shutterstock

Image 9: *Typical Cell Resting Within the Extracellular Matrix* by © Fran Kerg

Image 10: *Nerve Communication* - Public Domain

Image 11: *Chinese Finger Trap Toy* by Jose Gil - Shutterstock

Image 12: *Collagen Strand* by Studio Molekuul - Shutterstock

Image 13: *The Repetitive Cycle of Pain* by © Fran Kerg

Image 14: Jenga Puzzle by CHAMODZZ, Shutterstock

Image 15: *Pacinian Corpuscle* by © Fran Kerg

Image 16: *The Ion Channel* by W.Y.Sunshine - Shutterstock

Image 17: *Nerve Cell (Neuronal Anatomy)* by GraphicsRF.com - Shutterstock

Image 18: *The Sodium Potassium Pump* by Designa - Shutterstock

Image 19: *One Tendon Attaching Three Muscles to a Bone* by Andrea Danti – Shutterstock

Image 20: *Muscles Along the Spine* - Public Domain

Image 21: *Body Rotation for Moving Forward* by Dim Dimich - Shutterstock